W9-CEL-974

SKIN DEEP

Women on Skin Care, Makeup,

AND

Looking Their Best

The New York Times

BEE SHAPIRO

Principal Photography BY ELIZABETH LIPPMAN

02

04 Preface

07 Anna Kendrick

12 *Christophe Robin:*
On Iconic Blondes

14 Martha Stewart

19 *Best Lip Balms*

20 Alek Wek

26 *Pat McGrath: On the*
Influence of Fashion
on Beauty

28 Emily Ratajkowski

33 *DIY Tricks*

34 Stephanie Gilmore

40 Jenna Lyons

44 Ellie Goulding

48 Nina Dobrev

54 *Rachel Goodwin:*
On Camera-Ready
Skin That Looks
Beautiful in Real Life

56 Emily Weiss

62 Laure Heriard Dubreuil

66 Elle Macpherson

70 *Patrick Ta: How to Perfect*
Modern Smoky Eyes

73 *Lashing Out*

74 Patricia Clarkson

78 Rachel Roy

82 Julie Kent

88 Kylie Jenner

93 *Mario Dedivanovic:*
Social Media's Influence
on Beauty

96 Juliette Lewis

100 Julie de Libran

104 Karla Souza

109 *Covering Your Bases*

110 Natalia Vodianova

115 *Alexi Lubomirski: Behind*
the Scenes of Beauty
Photography

118 Emma Roberts

123 *Amy Wechsler: The*
Psychology of Wearing
Makeup to Work

124 Nicole Richie

128 Bobbi Brown

134 Priyanka Chopra

138 *Kira Nasrat: How to Do Bold, Believable Brows*

140 Skylar Diggins

144 Charli XCX

148 Isabel Toledo

152 Lisa Bonet

157 *Vive La France!*

158 Zoë Kravitz

162 *Rose-Marie Swift: How to Contour and Highlight like a Fashion Pro*

164 Lexi Boling

168 Jill Kargman

172 *Patricia Wexler: On Botox and Aging*

174 Zhu Zhu

180 Natalie Dormer

184 St. Vincent

190 Allyson Felix

194 Shala Monroque

199 *Pamela Neal: On Rock-and-Roll Hair*

202 Diane Kruger

207 *Taking the Highlighting Road*

208 Gwyneth Paltrow

213 *Serge Normant: On a Career in Celebrity Hair*

216 Jen Atkin

220 Madison Keys

226 *Dr. Dennis Gross: How to Maintain Clear Skin for an Active Lifestyle*

228 Sydney Sierota

232 Gabrielle Union-Wade

238 *Dendy Engelman: The New Methods of Achieving Celebrity Skin*

240 Brittany Snow

244 Molly Ringwald

249 *Power Lips*

250 Lily Collins

254 Acknowledgments

255 Index

Preface

Writing for a newspaper about what someone does to enhance her (or his) appearance can be a funny thing. Compared to wars, politics, and NASA breakthroughs, the topic might seem as frivolous as a ruffle on a dress. But it actually has tremendous depth, and I've come to love it for its—pardon the expression—many faces. Sure, there's the sheer thrill of the aesthetic (there are few daily things more pleasing than opening and closing a thoughtfully designed luxury compact). But I've also found it to be surprisingly inclusive and universal.

Though often thought of as aspirational, beauty—or rather the process of doing something to make oneself look, and therefore feel, better—is something anyone can achieve.

Even if some women prefer a less-is-more makeup routine, I have yet to meet a person, male or female, who doesn't desire flawless skin. Or perhaps someone has a streamlined skin care regimen but changing her hair color and style is more her thing.

From my interviews over the years, appearance is also incredibly intimate. Ask an actress what she's wearing on the red carpet and she'll happily divulge. But who did she go to for her subtle Botox? She'll likely balk or deny. Some of that secretive instinct is waning with the sharing (and oversharing) that's happening on social media, but I've found that it is far more difficult to convince celebrities to participate in an in-depth beauty interview than in a fashion column. They simply don't want to be seen as vain.

Which brings me to another lesson I've learned from covering this subject. Of course things like foundation and mascara are extraneous vanities, but the brighter side is that those little routines we do every morning and night are also a way for many people (myself included) to take care of themselves—and that's a good thing. Dedicating those few extra minutes can bring self-confidence and empowerment, and it can even dictate how we feel the rest of the day. Good hair day anyone?

It's this psychological effect that a good physical appearance has on us that continues to intrigue me. Full disclosure: A few years ago, I launched my own fragrance and body-care company, Ellis Brooklyn, which obviously entailed learning about practical facets of the business. But more intriguing was noticing how something like fragrance can trigger a rainbow of emotions and memories.

Which brings me to this book. Calling upon my interview notes and my memories has been a particular source of pleasure in putting together these pages. The celebrity interviews here span years, and they catch various women in many phases of their lives and careers. In broad strokes, wisdom about looking good is gained through experience. There are those, like Martha Stewart, Jenna Lyons, and Patricia Clarkson, who are so assured of their routine that their confidence and sense of humor radiates through the printed words. Others, like Emma Roberts, Madison Keys, and Kylie Jenner, are still in the process of discovery, and the joy they find in trial and error reveals something of their state of mind. And that's how beauty can be a disarming conversation starter, because it offers a different way to relay personality. Anna Kendrick may be all clever wit in most interviews, but who knew she was such a serious fragrance fan?

Certainly appearance is often manipulated in film and on stage to create character. So in real life, does it say something about you? My first job out of school was as a hedge fund attorney in Midtown Manhattan. As a mid-twentysome-thing in a room full of older men, my armor was my slick black liquid liner, rose-brown lips, and a manicure I ran out to get professionally done every single week. I'll never know if the look actually lent me any authority, but at the time I felt it gave me more of a take-me-seriously appeal.

I started writing Skin Deep for the Style Pages of *The New York Times* in my mid- to late-twenties, when I was single and could go out until 1 A.M. on a weekday without major repercussions in the morning. Now I am a decade older and married with two little ones whose love for waking up at the crack of dawn can make the slightest hangover painful. You can say I grew up with the column over the years.

While the articles in this collection aren't strictly relegated to celebrities, it's undeniable that they have played an incredibly influential role, and the interviews with famous and notable women on their regimens seem to have struck a chord with readers. Here are women who otherwise appeared out of reach, sitting down at their vanities and sharing the same joys, insecurities, and triumphs anyone might feel. I've arranged the interviews here to provide variety and contrast—perhaps a serious beauty devotee followed by a regimen minimalist, or a paragon of high culture before a social media darling. So as you read through the pages of this book, I hope you're able not only to take away some useful tips and learn about new products, but to also see another side to these well-known women. But mostly, I hope you'll enjoy the ride. After all, the politics and wars will still be there. This? This is fun.

Anna Kendrick

Actress and Author

FRAGRANCE

I like to buy a new fragrance for each film. I'll go out in the city where I'm filming and snap it up. It's not really intentional; it kind of has to find you. The one that I have for *Into the Woods* is Terry de Gunzburg Flagrant Délice, which I bought in London. But the one that I'm wearing now is Orange Flower & Lychee by Kiehl's, which is from *Happy Christmas*. I was feeling nostalgic. That's the thing about fragrance, memory is so attached. I also love buying fragrance for special times in my life. Like maybe if I got engaged, I'd buy one.

SKIN CARE

I do this AKMD foaming face wash, which no one has ever heard of, but it's awesome if your skin is a little bit oily. I honestly don't know where it came from. It just ended up in my bathroom cabinet. Then I do the SK-II Facial Treatment Essence, which is like a toner. I feel like I turn over a new layer of skin every time I use it, which I need because I travel so much. I always end up breaking out when I fly a lot, but I've realized the most important thing when traveling is being moisturized. So now I'm using the Kate Somerville Nourish Daily Moisturizer. Sometimes I'll throw on a Kate Somerville eye cream, but most of the time, I'm too lazy. I'm really into lip oil though. I have this one by Hourglass—it's an oil with this gold-tip applicator and it's schmancy-schmancy. It's because I'm so fancy; I've got to keep it glossy. No really, when you get to the point that your lips are cracking, the price is worth it.

Let me tell you, my sunscreen is the best. It's the Aveeno Smart Essentials moisturizer with SPF 30. I hate the way sunscreen smells; it always reminds me of being a kid, all sticky at the beach. This one just smells like lotion.

Oh, and if you're not using Schick Intuition razors, you're wasting everybody's time. It cuts your shower time in half. Whenever I hear somebody is still using a separate shave gel (the Intuition has it in the razor), it's like hearing they still use dial-up Internet.

At night, it's pretty much the same stuff. Although, I just found the best wipes. You know how wipes make your skin feel tight and sticky but you're too lazy to actually go wash your face? Not this one. It's by Koh Gen Do. Again, it's not cheap, but so, so worth it.

MAKEUP

I use Bobbi Brown foundation—the Long-Wear Even Finish one. I actually blend the 0 and the 3.25 shades together, because that's what my makeup artist did for *Into the Woods*. (It's much more fun playing dirty Cinderella because you can cover up any blemishes with tons of dirt.) I would not have thought to blend two colors that aren't side by side on the color spectrum, but it looks gorgeous.

I've started using NARS Contour Blush in Olympia. I was so scared of contour—you see photos of girls on Instagram with that shiny plastic, war-paint look—but this one is so subtle. For mascara, I use Guerlain Maxi Lash. It's a great mascara and all, but it actually smells really good too. It seems silly, but for a product you use every day, it's kind of a nice touch.

I'm obsessed with eyebrows. In my dreams, I have Keira Knightley's eyebrows. But it's just not in the cards for me, so I do what I can. I use this eyebrow liquid pen by this Japanese brand, Suqqu. I found it when I was in England. It is a game changer; you never ever get that starting blob of eyebrow that you get with your regular pencil or powder or whatever. It's impossible to mess up.

I'm not big on lip color, but I like to have a little bit of something. I just ordered a big size of Jane Iredale Just Kissed Lip and Cheek Stain. It doesn't just give you that bee-stung thing for two seconds; it lasts for hours.

HAIR

I haven't had a haircut in so long. I kind of just get it cut on set—that makes me sound cheap and lazy! At home, I'm using the Oribe Shampoo and Masque for Beautiful Color. My hair isn't colored right now, but I'm still feeling the repercussions from going blonde for a film last year. For styling, I use the Oribe Dry Texturizing Spray that everybody loves. I also use a Shu Uemura hair oil. I put it on before I blow dry. I feel like hair oils help a lot.

SERVICES

I find getting my nails done the most tedious thing. I'm such a fidgety person—it's like torture. I tried massages for my last movie because it was really physical, but again, I'm the worst person. Everybody loves massages;

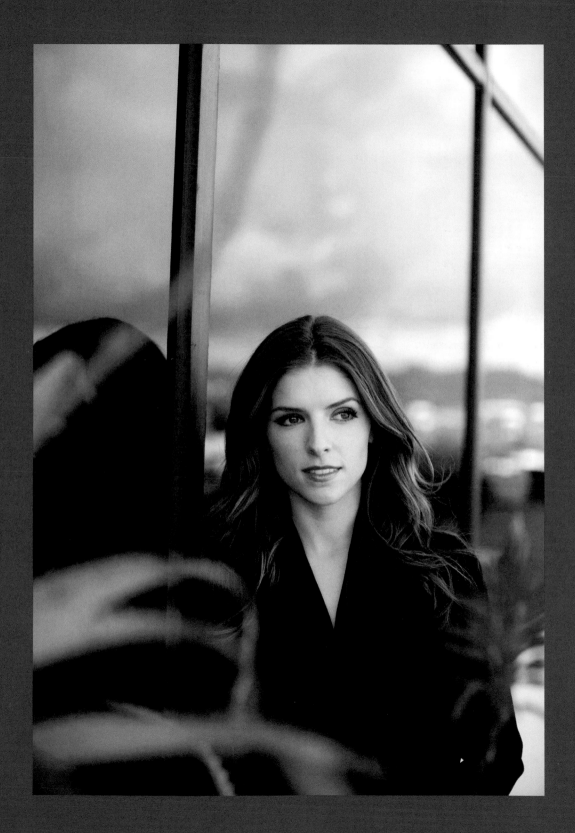

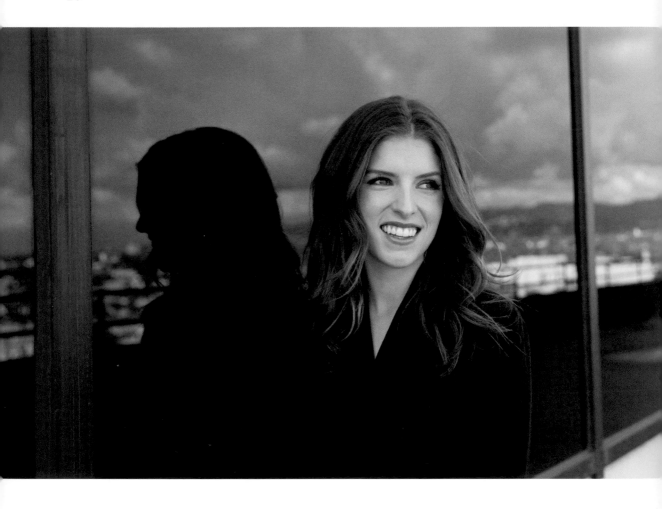

I don't know what my problem is. I feel like I have to talk to the masseuses. Pretty soon, I'm asking for their grandma's recipe for apple pie and pretending like I'm interested. Why? Besides, I'd rather do this face to face when their hands aren't all over my naked body.

DIET AND FITNESS

I feel like thirty is just around the corner, and I'm reluctantly trying to take care of myself. My friend Aubrey Plaza has been trying to get me to be a grown-up and to not eat the junk that I do. So I'm being dragged kicking and screaming into adulthood. Now I'm taking Pure Barre and eating fancy cereal with almond milk for breakfast. The most disappointing part is how great I feel. I even like this Daily Greens juice called Purity. It tastes like you're eating grass, but you feel so freaking good after it. I'm sure part of it is mental.

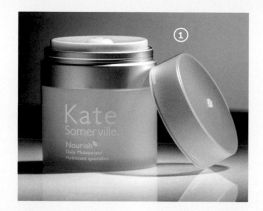

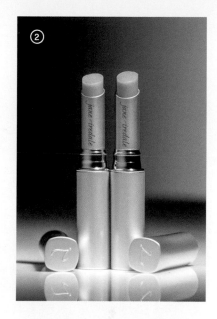

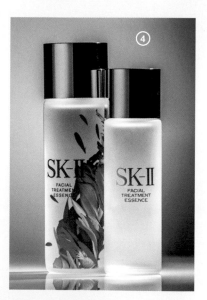

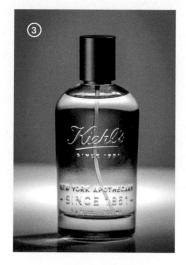

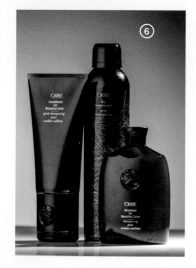

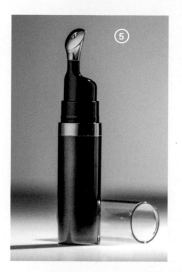

1 **Kate Somerville** Nourish Daily Moisturizer

2 **Jane Iredale** Just Kissed Lip and Cheek Stain

3 **Kiehl's** Orange Flower & Lychee

4 **SK-II** Facial Treatment Essence

5 **Hourglass** No. 28 Lip Treatment Oil

6 **Oribe** Shampoo and Conditioner for Beautiful Color, Dry Texturizing Spray

CHRISTOPHE ROBIN
ON ICONIC BLONDES

When I think of icy iconic blondes, I think of Catherine Deneuve in *Belle de Jour*. Though she's certainly moved on from this role, her blonde mane is still one of her signatures. The man behind her frosty shade? Paris-based hair colorist Christophe Robin, who has a knack for creating statement blondes that feel lively and real rather than flat and cartoonish. I also love how he approaches haircare. Sure, he has his own wonderful line—I particularly love his sea-salt hair scrub, which imparts divine texture for fine or stick-straight strands—but he also dishes practical advice anyone, not just famous actresses, can try. He's given me such simple, effective tips as washing my hair upside down (it boosts circulation, he says) to finishing my in-shower routine with a DIY diluted apple cider vinegar scalp rinse (it keeps the greasies away).

When did you start doing celebrities in your salon practice?
It was indeed straight away. I opened my first salon when I was twenty-four years old—it was dedicated to hair color only, which was really a unique concept at the time. At that point, I had already been working for quite some time and had the opportunity to evolve in the fashion world—I was coloring the supermodels at the time.

Supermodels then were certainly celebrities. Who was your first one?
When I first arrived in Paris, I used to work for one of the biggest salon franchises, Jean Louis David. He also owned studios on the side that were meant for ad campaign shoots. I remember this was at the very beginning of the supermodels, and someone from the team called me on a photo shoot because they could not make the model's hair shine. I was barely eighteen and did not know anything about fashion and had never heard about Stephanie Seymour until then! She ended up loving my work, and from that point on, it was like a snowball effect. Models realized we could play with color, therefore allowing them to play with their appearances. I remember this haute couture collection with Yves Saint Laurent where all the girls had extraordinary hair colors. Sibyl Buck had deep red hair, Alice Dodd blood orange hair . . . .

Is there a difference, from a coloring standpoint, between fashion and celebrity?
Coloring hair for a photo shoot or a film is different than coloring a celebrity who comes into my salon. There are a lot of things to take into consideration when shooting—lighting can be tricky and the result on camera is always different. You always have to work with those things in mind.

Putting aside supermodels for a minute, what do you think about the phenomenon that is "celebrity hair"?
Each time period has its opinion leaders. When I first started, it was the supermodels. Then it

became the actresses who started appearing more and more on magazine covers. Today, it clearly revolves around influencers—bloggers and reality TV personalities.

Celebrity still makes quite a lasting impact though. You're particularly known for your work with Catherine Deneuve. How did that come about?

She called me one day at my salon; she had seen Claudia Schiffer's blonde and loved it and wanted to know who was behind it. Ever since, she has been coming to me for her color and, over time, has even helped me develop some of my products. I always ask for her input and feedback—she really is an expert and passionate about beauty. Also, Catherine has a blonde that evolves with her movies and roles. But it always involves contrast to brighten up her eyes.

What do you mean by contrast?

It's important that the color complements the complexion—not all blondes are the same. The color depends on the skin tone, color of the eyes … in the end it has to look natural and your hair has to feel and look healthy.

To me, that sounds like the whole French hair thing that many American women are after. What's the secret?

French hair is meant to be effortless and low-maintenance. In terms of color, it's the same. French hair is about more natural colors with a lot of contrasts, meaning chestnuts with no warm tones.

CHRISTOPHE ROBIN'S BLOND HAIR MISTAKES TO AVOID

Not Protecting Your Hair Before Highlighting: There's a plethora of hair bond strengtheners (think Olaplex) used during the hair-dying process that have changed the coloring game—that is, even bleached blondes have significantly healthier strands. But Christophe starts hydrating hair *before* any chemicals are applied. "I usually apply my Moisturizing Hair Oil with Lavender before any color process," he says. "It really protects the hair and allows the color to last longer."

Streaks: Unless you're purposely going for a skunk look, Christophe says, "contrasts should be subtle to make it look more natural."

Going Too Blonde: Blonde ambition much? Christophe sees this as a common mistake. The blonde should match your complexion, he says. "If you have very dark eyes, it's important to keep a little bit of your natural color at the roots to create some contrast."

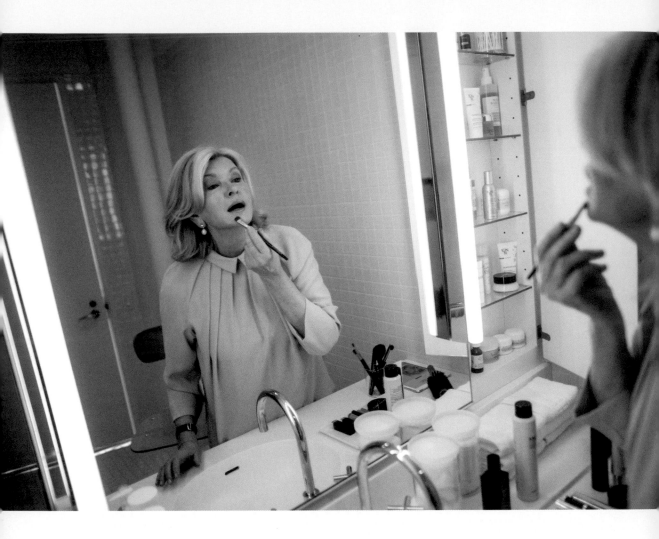

Martha Stewart

TV Personality, Author,

and Entrepreneur

SKIN CARE

I get up a couple of hours before I'm supposed to leave in the morning and I'll put on a mask. I like the Yon-Ka Gommage 305 or the Susan Ciminelli Hydrating Gel Mask right now. Or I'll use the Super Collagen Mask from Mario Badescu or the Chanel Ultra Correction Lift, a firming mask, which works great for me. I'll do this about five days a week, and I don't repeat the same mask two days in a row. I've always done this—well, basically since I discovered masks. I have to wear makeup for photo shoots, television, and appearances, so I have to make sure my face is extremely clean in the morning. Then I shower and I wash it all off.

I slather myself with serums. First, it's a toning lotion. Right now it's either the Yon-Ka lotion or a more specific spray, like the rosewater

Facial Spray from Mario Badescu. I spray my whole face and body and then it's Susan Ciminelli Marine Lotion from head to toe. I use the same products on my body as I use on my face. I don't think there's really any difference between the two, so the more moisturizers and serums you use, the better off you are. Then I might use a vitamin B or SkinCeuticals C E Ferulic serum. I'll also put on Clé de Peau or SkinCeuticals moisturizer. With all of these serums, I find I don't have to put on an eye cream, although my facialist insists I put one on. Sometimes I will, and the Clé de Peau is good, or Caudalie has one—it's the fancy one from their high-end line—and it's very good too. At the end, before any makeup, I use SkinCeuticals Physical Fusion UV Defense. If I'm not going to use foundation, I'll use the tinted version, or if I use foundation, it'll be the white one. Otherwise, I do my best to stay out of the sun. That's very important. I do a lot of outdoor activity, like gardening, and I try to cover up and use SPF. Actually, I just bought a new sun hat that goes over your riding helmet. It's pretty ugly, but it works.

If I'm traveling, I'll be sure to have my Yon-Ka lotion with me, which is a spray. On a recent plane ride to L.A., I sprayed myself five times. It's hydrating, so I don't look like a prune after flying.

I never go to bed with makeup on. First, I steam my face with a hot washcloth, and then I use AmorePacific or Shu Uemura cleansing oils. Johnson's baby oil works really well too. I use those as cleansers, and they're also excellent makeup removers. I like oil because it keeps my skin very moist, and it works for me. I don't get clogged pores.

MAKEUP

I was told years ago by my daughter Alexis that I shouldn't leave the house without makeup on. You'll pay for it if you do, because somebody will be there with a camera snapping away and you'll look awful or just plain. I put on a light foundation, usually the AmorePacific tube called the Moisture Bound Tinted Treatment Moisturizer or the Clé de Peau Refining Fluid Foundation. I really like the YSL Touche Éclat radiant touch stick. Then it's Bobbi Brown bronzer. For mascara, I use Clinique High Impact Mascara or I just got a new one from Givenchy. The wand has three little balls almost—it's very cute. I got it from a makeup artist at John Barrett, when she did my eyes for the ballet. It's a little short mascara wand, but it makes your eyelashes look elongated. Also, I've used Latisse and it's really helped. People should try that. It really works. I use a gloss on my lips. I use Buxom—I like the Samantha color—or a little bit of a lip pencil. I stick with nude colors, and maybe at night, I'll wear red and it'll really stand out.

FRAGRANCE

I've been wearing Fracas since I was nineteen. I'll put fragrance on three times a day. I'm thankful every day that they haven't altered their formula. Although, I did just discover a new one by Hermès called Jour D'Hermès. It's lovely.

HAIR

I use different shampoos. For me, it's like with skin care: I try to use a variety. I have to wash my hair almost every day because I have to have it done for pictures and stuff. Frédéric Fekkai Ageless Rejuvenating Shampoo and Restructuring Conditioner and Shu Uemura, the green line, are my favorites. For styling, I don't like a lot of mousse. I do use Sally Hershberger Salon Texture Blast, which is like a hair spray, but just at the roots. I have really good hair and I don't like to plaster it.

Parvin at John Barrett has been my colorist forever. She's the blonde expert. I think she's the busiest colorist in New York. I like her because she does it in an hour so you don't have to spend all day sitting there.

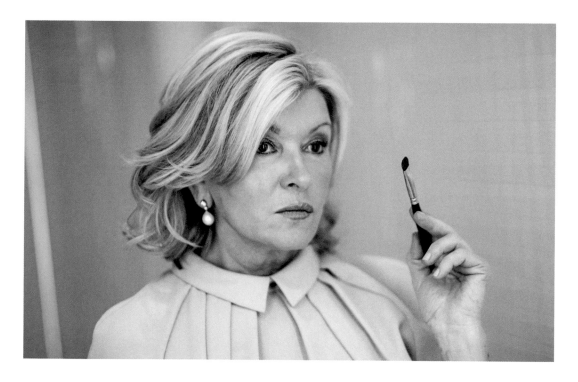

For cuts, I'm not fussy. I've been to Kevin at Frédéric Fekkai in The Mark Hotel. I've gotten my hair cut twice at Sally Hershberger recently and they're fabulous too. There are so many fantastic haircutters in the city. Everybody's hair looks much better than it used to.

Otherwise, Daisy Schwartzberg does my daily makeup and styling. Kevin from Fekkai will do styling for photo shoots and Katsu from John Barrett does my blowout. They're all good.

SERVICES

I've been going to Mario Badescu for facials for forty-five years. I try to go at least once a month. For brows, there's a fabulous Russian girl at John Barrett who does them when I get my hair done. Luda, also at John Barrett—where else in New York can you get everything done at once?—does my nails almost exclusively. And she's the best massager in the world. I stand, walk, and hike and I still have good feet, and I thank her for that.

DIET AND FITNESS

Exercise is a necessary part of the day. I went to the gym this morning. I have a really great trainer in the city. We've worked together for at least eight years. Or I do yoga with James Murphy. I like to spin, but I don't have enough time to do it. I also have a green juice that I drink every single morning. It's very important. You can be the most beautiful person on earth and if you don't have a fitness or diet routine, you won't be beautiful.

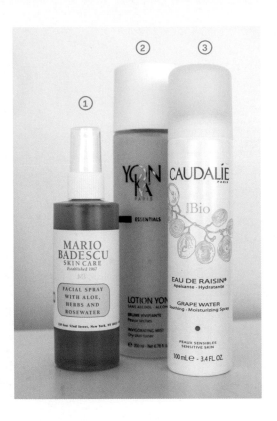

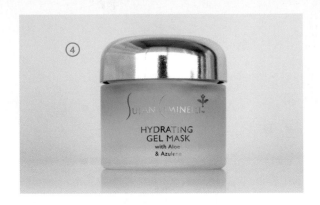

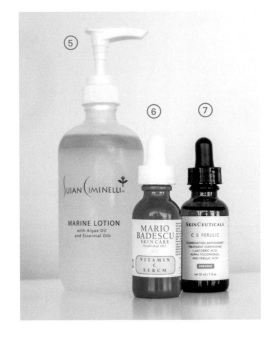

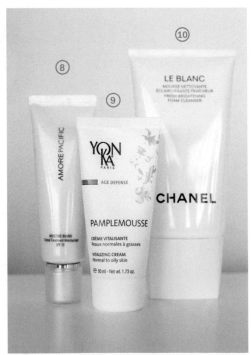

1   **Mario Badescu**
Facial Spray

2   **Yon-Ka**
Lotion Yon-Ka

3   **Caudalíe**
Grape Water

4   **Susan Ciminelli**
Hydrating Gel Mask

5   **Susan Ciminelli**
Marine Lotion

6   **Mario Badescu**
Vitamin C Serum

7   **SkinCeuticals**
C E Ferulic serum

8   **AmorePacific**
Moisture Bound
Tinted Treatment
Moisturizer

9   **Yon-Ka**
Pamplemousse
Vitalizing Cream

10   **Chanel** Le Blanc
Foam Cleanser

BEST LIP BALMS

For anyone ever addicted to lip balm, here are a few highlights.

NUXE RÊVE DE MIEL

I first spotted this backstage at a fashion show where Pat McGrath was running makeup. She was prepping each model's lips with this little pot before applying lipstick. It offers a nice balance of hydration and staying power, but perhaps best of all for lip-product wearers, the finish is a sophisticated demi-matte. No slick messes from lip balm here.

HOURGLASS NO. 28 LIP TREATMENT OIL

With the gold tip applicator, "it's schmancy-schmancy," says Anna Kendrick. "It's because I'm so fancy; I've got to keep it glossy. No really, when you get to the point that your lips are cracking, the price is worth it."

SMITH'S ROSEBUD SALVE

Lily Collins throws this one in her bag. "I always wear lip balm. I'm constantly reapplying."

AQUAPHOR

Drew Barrymore says she "can't live without" this staple. (Kylie Jenner and Emily Ratajkowski are also fans.) It's also multipurpose—it works wonders on chapped lips or irritated winter skin.

BURT'S BEES

Juliette Lewis prefers her balms on the natural side. She picks up this beauty editor favorite at Whole Foods.

KIEHL'S EUCALYPTUS LIP RELIEF

Model Alek Wek enjoys Kiehl's entire eucalyptus line for its zingy fresh effect.

LUCAS' PAPAW OINTMENT

Nicole Richie likes her balm so much, she uses it in this unique way: "I'll also stick it up my nose with a Q-tip when I fly, so I don't get sick," she says. "It works."

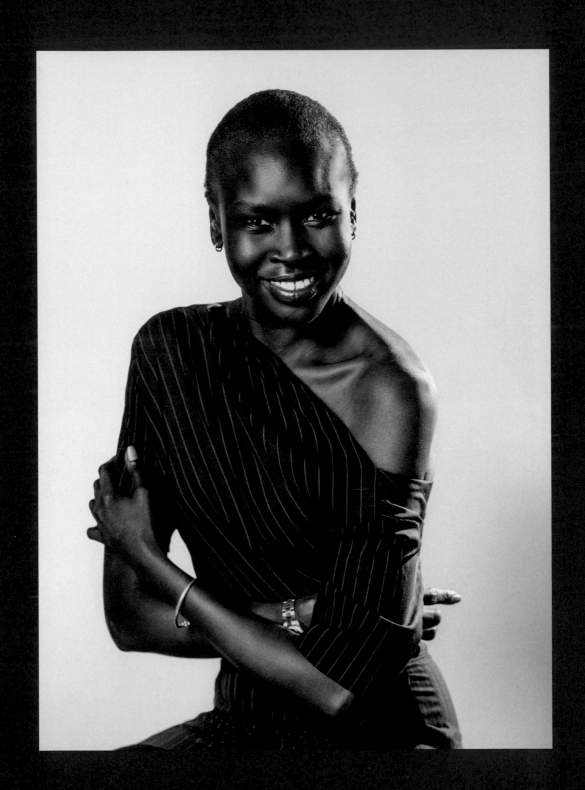

Alek Wek

Model

MAKEUP

When I got into this business, it was the '90s. There wasn't anybody working who had my features—who I could relate to. People in this business try to compare you. If you're a new girl, they'd say, "Oh, she's like a baby Cindy," or "She looks like the next Kate Moss."

With me, they might say, "Oh she looks like Grace Jones," but she's a completely different woman.

I made it through the beginning because of what my mother embedded in us. She had nine of us and five are girls. She always said, we have to support each other. "Together you are stronger. You're beautiful inside and out." Still, it was so challenging.

I'll never forget my first spread though. It was for Italian *Vogue* with Steven Meisel and there were all these Versace dresses. This was right before Gianni Versace passed away. Steven put

on the music and he said, "Alek, just go." I was like nineteen or twenty and I started dancing and I was like, "Yes! I can be just Alek." That was a moment where I came alive. I thought, "OK, I can do this. I can just be Alek and make it in this industry." I knew that whatever young girl out there, who would grow up, could look at me, and might think, "It's OK to be you. It's OK to be shy. It's OK to not know if you're not sure about something."

I'm glad we're moving toward that in fashion, because the world is truly a rainbow. Fashion draws so much inspiration from different countries and cultures. We should be representing more of what the population actually looks like. We can do this change individually, whether it's an agent who really works on behalf of the girls—the clients or the girls themselves. The girls have to really want to be themselves.

As they say, though, the proof is in the

pudding. Pull out the range of foundation colors of a brand and you can see it. They're not serving all these women out there.

If I'm not working, I try to not wear anything on my skin. The best makeup and concealer is getting eight hours of sleep and a good steam.

If I do put on makeup, MAC has foundation colors that work for my skin. When I first started working, there were no colors that suited me. There wasn't all this variation we have today, so when I saw great colors on women, I would stop them and say, "Wow, where did you get that?"

I'm girly inside: I love a little shimmer on my eyes and on my cheeks. When you wear something you like, it does make you feel good and reflects your mood. L'Oréal has some that are quite fun, and I also like the Revlon shimmers that come in a round container. I even use it on my arms and my legs during the summer.

The Juicy Tubes by Lancôme are so good. I'm like the queen of those. Sometimes they put glitter in them, which is even better.

My skin has a little purple in it. I love a little blush by YSL—they have a nice orange, and I also like the ones with a little bit of red and purple. Shu Uemura is very good with their powders. They have a white powder that goes on clear and it works on everybody. That's one of those tips I picked up from being on shoots.

For lip colors, the NARS Times Square, which is a dark aubergine, has always worked on me.

I'm not big on drawing eyebrows. But I do love fake lashes. Shu Uemura has really nice ones—I can put them on myself. And I love me a good mascara. Again, I like Shu Uemura, and YSL also has a great one that I tried from a goodie bag.

SKIN CARE

When I wake up, I use warm water and Dove soap to wash—it's really gentle. Then I brush, floss, and shower, and then apply moisturizer everywhere. My favorite is by John-son's—it's the baby oil gel and comes in a bunch of different varieties. I like the chamomile and the shea and cocoa butter ones. Johnson's is very mild as well. Running around the shows and doing shoots, you use a lot of products. So I try to not use anything harsh if it's just my own time.

Sometimes, I'll switch to Kiehl's. I use the Lip Relief with eucalyptus and the body cream, which I use on my face as well.

And the good thing with working with the lovely teams that make us look wonderful and glamorous for fashion shoots is that you pick up tips. There was one cream that one person on set couldn't stop talking about and pretty soon literally everyone had to have it. That would be Embryolisse Lait-Crème Concentré . I use it on my face and it's fantastic. It used to be hard to get. I pick up four tubes whenever I'm in Paris.

I do put on sunscreen. Nivea has one that I was spray-ing on. I also use it for my face. I put it on my hands and then pat it on. And I'll wear a hat, which I love to do, but it's also for the protection.

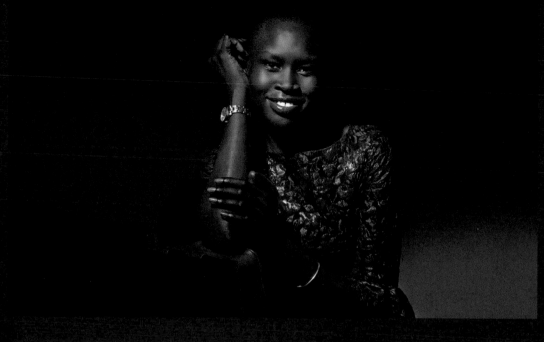
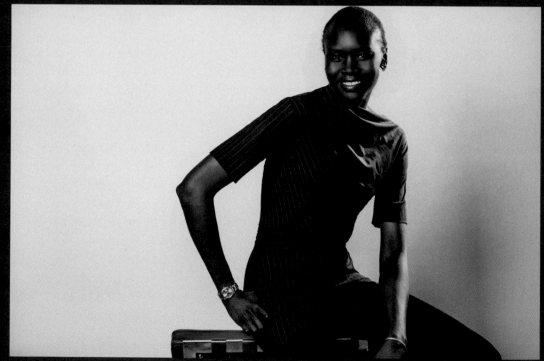

If I do a shoot and they put makeup around my eyes and do the eyelashes and all that, then of course you can't just wash your face and go to sleep. You might get an eye infection. The Lancôme Bi-Facil is really good. It never lets you down.

HAIR

I've kept my hair short—no longer than three to four inches—and I like to fade it in the back. It fits my face shape and it's also easy because it's wash-and-go as well. In the summer, if I go on a holiday, then I do cornrows. I have them done in Brooklyn by a lovely lady on Jay Street.

It's really boring, but I use Johnson's baby shampoo. My hair is very thin—like baby hair. I'm really scared to use a harsh shampoo. Then I use a lot, a lot of conditioner. I like the Aveda Brilliant one.

FRAGRANCE

I love fragrance. My favorite notes are lavender and vetiver. I used to be very into the Acqua di Parma scents. Now I'm back to my old favorite, the Hermès Bel Ami Vetiver scent, which is a little unisex. For me, vetiver brings back memories. Where I come from, when you have a baby, you have a baby shower. Then, after the woman stays in for forty days after giving birth, they slaughter a goat and they make sandalwood incense and this oil that smells of vetiver. This has stuck with me.

I also like to try new things though. One of my new ones is Decadence by Marc Jacobs. It's an evening scent and just smells yummy.

OTHER SERVICES

A sauna or steam room really opens my skin. I literally look rejuvenated. Even the simple places are terrific. I'll go to the steam room at Equinox—I'm a member—and I might do a massage there too. Soho Sanctuary is very good for massages as well.

DIET AND FITNESS

I do yoga every morning. I drag my mat everywhere with me. The older you get, the more you need to stretch. The way I started, I was reading the Dalai Lama books, believe it or not. It triggered something in me. I was reading about how it makes you be comfortable with your body and the benefits from it, and I thought, "This is for me!" This was eight years ago, but just to clarify, I'm still an amateur.

In terms of weight, I don't really pay attention to that—knock on wood. It's a genetic thing. I did try to be vegetarian for a while, but that was not good for me. Now I eat everything, but I do a lot of dark green vegetables and lots of fish, which really helps my skin. I also do a lot of home cooking—that way I know what is going in my food. I tried to grow stuff—herbs and vegetables—in my garden at home in Brooklyn, but the squirrels got to them! Right now, I just do flowers in the garden, but one of these days, I'll grow vegetables.

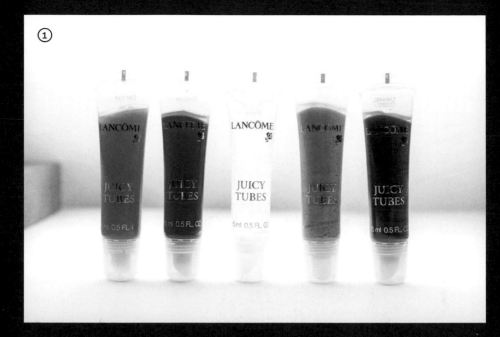

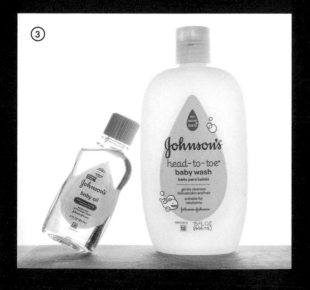

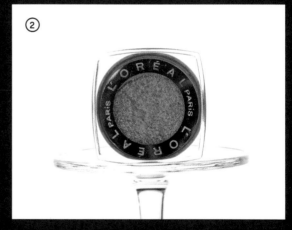

1 **Lancôme**
Juicy Tubes

2 **L'Oréal**
Shimmer Powder

3 **Johnson's**
Baby Oil, Baby Wash

PAT MCGRATH
ON THE
INFLUENCE OF
FASHION ON BEAUTY

Pat McGrath is considered by many to be the greatest makeup artist working today. I first witnessed her vivacious and dominating personality at 8 A.M. on a Sunday at New York Fashion Week. It was an early call time by fashion week standards, and though it was for the Victoria Beckham runway show and Victoria, David, and their kids were all there, it was McGrath who wholly commanded the attention of her team with her precise application and quips capped with "Darling!" "Gorgeous!" "Fabulous!" Her work can be subtle and beautiful, but it's her divine and playful interpretations of glamour—crystal-encrusted lips and spider lashes never looked so good—that I'm constantly tracking. These days, she's channeling her charismatic energies into her own cosmetics line, which is targeted to her fellow makeup obsessives.

When did you fall in love with beauty?
I've loved makeup since I was six or seven. My mother was obsessed with cosmetics and therefore I was obsessed with cosmetics. I knew one day, like many little girls who watched their moms put on their makeup, that I was going to snatch that lipstick off the table for myself.

What were your early influences?
Mine was really from my mother talking about what she wanted. She was obsessed with textures and finding certain colors. After that, when I was older, I was influenced by music from David Bowie to Marc Bolan. Then it was the New Romantics, Leigh Bowery, Grace Jones, and all of that.

Having made your career in fashion, have you seen its influence on beauty change over the years?
To me, it's very much the same, which is the fact that everything changes constantly all of the time. One moment, it's fashion that is dictating the look. Or you can get an influence from a film. Other times, you might see something in a movie but fashion has infiltrated into the look. I think that's the joy and the brilliance of fashion and beauty. And now with social media, we're just constantly being bombarded with genius imagery that inspires us every second.

Speaking of social media, there are some established artists of your generation who aren't as keen on what's happening in beauty on Instagram, etc. How do you see it?

For me, social media is amazing. For years and years, you worked in a very closed circle—that was fashion. So outside of the industry, of course, no one really knows who you are. But then I remember the first time I went onto Twitter. It was thanks to the lovely Coco Rocha; she helped me create an account. Once I signed on, there were thousands of people saying "Hi" or even talking about work I did ten years ago. They would say things like, "Oh those Swarovski lips or spidery lashes you did—that really affected me." Hearing that—it was an incredible day. Later, it became also about being able to look at young artists and the work they were doing.

Do you think with the rise of social media, people are more willing to wear editorial looks?
Yes, they are. People are realizing editorial is actually more wearable in a way. We've never done 90-point contouring on faces for editorials. That's what you're seeing on Instagram. For the runway, that would be a mess. So people are seeing that when you're talking about a runway look, there's more modernity, freshness, and wearability. If you're talking about a glitter lip, don't wear it with twenty tons of mascara. Why not try it with a fresh face? It brings a whole new view on the idea of makeup as an accessory. And women are not afraid of trying the runway look, because they've been struggling to do a 90-point fake contour. She can apply the glitter lip and that's like nothing to her. Today's beauty customer is a lot more informed and skilled.

What are some of your favorite beauty looks you've created over the years?
I've always been the one to really push boundaries. I think of the Swarovski crystal masks and crystal lips, and also the paper eyeliner I've done. I remember the first time I did very clumpy eyelashes for John Galliano at Dior. I think it made the cover of a newspaper: They said women wouldn't wear them. Of course, that's the norm now.

One thing that's always been important to me, though, is really glowing skin. It's figuring out how to contour the face with light. Now they call it "strobing." But at one point, some people were saying skin had to be matte and perfect. Those are the rules I love to challenge.

Are there certain models who really know how to work makeup? There are so many. It's really about being able to convey emotion, and some models are almost like great actresses in their pictures. Definitely Kristen McMenamy, Naomi Campbell, Amber Valletta, Linda Evangelista, Jamie Bochert, and Guinevere van Seenus are like that. Ajak Deng, she's also fabulous. They bring more than just a pretty face.

Where do you get inspiration for your work?
That's something I do almost every day: I'm looking for something I've never seen before. That's my obsession. What works magnificently but gives us an otherworldly finish? Inspiration is in every walk of life. I can be inspired by everything from art to movies to the vintage books I buy.

Emily Ratajkowski

Actress and Social Media Star

MAKEUP

There are so many unique actresses in the industry now that there's a lot more acceptance of what's considered beautiful. I probably have more of an editorial or model-y look, but then I have an L.A. body. I also can work my look so it's more on the pretty side of things, which is what they like in L.A. But in general, it's just hard to be a young woman in Hollywood. It doesn't matter what your look is or what you want to accomplish. It's a crazy world of men trying to fit women into boxes. I couldn't believe it when I first started working in the industry, but it truly is still such a boys' club. Even so, I haven't let that affect my choices in beauty. You just have to do what feels good for yourself and not apologize for it.

I have really big features, so a little makeup goes a long way. I would hate to look like a clown. During the day, I use the Glossier Perfecting Skin Tint; I'm using the dark color because I have a bit of a tan right now. I'm not sure it really covers much, but it just evens me out. Then I'll use the

Charlotte Tilbury mascara and cream blush. Charlotte provided all the makeup for *We Are Your Friends*, so that's how I got to try all her products. Then I put Aquaphor on my lips and just let that be or I might mix it with Charlotte's Bond Girl Matte Revolution Lipstick so there's some definition. I have really pale lips—people always think I'm wearing nude lipstick.

If I have a meeting or need to look more done-up, the thing I can always do is a cat eye. I like the Revlon ColorStay liner. I have a comb for my eyebrows that I spray with Elnett. And I'm really loving Charlotte's Filmstar Bronze & Glow, which has a highlighter and a contour shade. I only use the highlighter, though. I put it on the top of my cheekbones, down the line of my nose, and on my Cupid's bow. I'm not big on contouring; my features are really out there already.

SKIN CARE

I have the same skin care routine morning and night, although I'm not one of those people

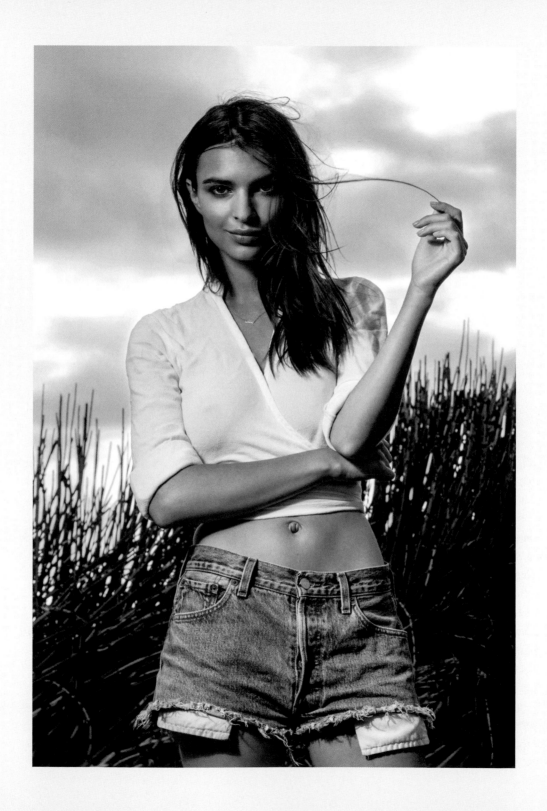

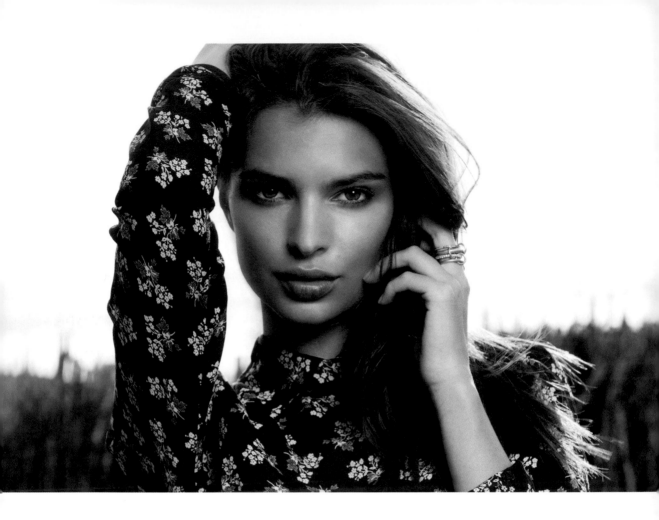

who always uses the same products. My skin changes with the weather. Right now I'm using Kiehl's Calendula Deep Cleansing Foaming Face Wash. Then I brush my teeth and I put on moisturizer. The By Terry Cellularose Baume D'Eau is great. A lot of moisturizers, they don't absorb into your skin quickly enough, but this one seeps in right away. I also like the Sisley Paris Hydra-Global—it smells so good. If I need makeup remover, I use this L'Oreal eye makeup remover that my mom introduced me to years ago. At night, I might add on the Sisley Paris Black Rose Precious Face Oil, which is also about the smell—this gorgeous rose.

When I'm traveling, though, I'll bring along my Glossier Mega Greens Galaxy Pack. It's a mask, and I put it on after a flight. That's one of my favorite things to do: When I get to the hotel, I put it on for twenty minutes and my skin feels so much better. Of course, you have to drink a lot of water in the air, but here's another one of my favorites: If it's a long flight, I'll wash my face before sleeping and put on the Sisley Paris Express Flower Gel. It's a mask that you don't have to wash off—it's perfect for the plane.

FRAGRANCE

I actually don't wear fragrance. Even my body lotion, by Bliss, is unscented. I always feel like I smell cheap. I guess I just haven't smelled one that's not too overpowering or too sweet. Or even when I try one of the super masculine scents, I just think, "I don't want to smell like a man." Besides, I like my own scent.

HAIR

I shower every other day. Right now, I'm kind of in-between shampoos and conditioners. But I was just in Positano for vacation and stayed at this place called Le Sirenuse; they have their own shampoo and conditioner. I took home four bottles, but they're already starting to dwindle. They smell amazing. I'm going to have to reorder.

I put my hair up maybe half the time—parted down the middle and maybe slicked, Dolce & Gabbana style. When my hair is down, it's very straight. I try to add a little volume with Bumble and bumble dry shampoo and then part it down the middle. Sometimes, when it's too straight, I'll curl the ends and maybe a little around the back of the head so it has a little bit of volume. It usually falls quickly, but it's nice to try. I like my Conair wand—it's a drugstore find.

OTHER SERVICES

I'm pretty terrified of facials. I've had enough bad ones, and honestly, I don't break out. So it's a "Why mess with a good thing?" kind of deal. My big treat is going to the Korean spa once a month. The one I go to, called Natura, is a little less popular than the ones most of Hollywood goes to. I usually go about forty minutes before my appointment, and you can get into all these different types of pools. Then you get a body scrub and you're lying there naked with twenty other women out there! They just treat you like a piece of meat, but it's worth it.

Then you shower, and my hair is down, it's very straight. I like the acupressure massage—those ladies are strong! They even put grated cucumber on your face. I do have to warn that it's not your traditional spa. There is no one greeting you and asking how your day is. But that's what I love about it. You totally shut off, and that's what I'm looking for. I want to completely relax, let my mind shut off, and have someone take care of what needs to be done. Afterward, my skin is so soft, and I always sleep so well that night.

DIET AND FITNESS

I'm very lucky. With me, a little goes a long way. It's about feeling good about what you eat. I do love turmeric and beet juices. It's just so L.A., you can't even avoid it. But I don't have a trainer, and I don't really go to the gym. I go on long walks and hikes with my girlfriends. That's about it. I'm just not a crazy fitness person. I'm definitely an outlier in the industry.

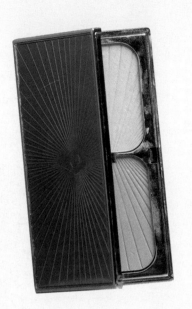

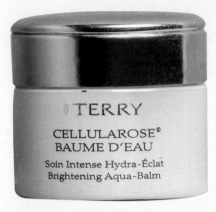

① ② ③ ④ ⑤

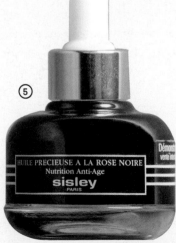

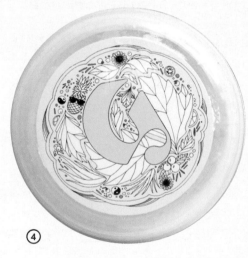

1	**Charlotte Tilbury** Filmstar Bronze & Glow	3	**Revlon** ColorStay liner
2	**By Terry** Cellularose Baume D'Eau	4	**Glossier** Mega Greens Galaxy Pack
		5	**Sisley Paris** Black Rose Precious Face Oil

DIY TRICKS

Who doesn't love a little do-it-yourself beauty trick? It's the wisdom passed down through generations of women.

HONEY MASK

"If I ever get a sunburn, I'll put honey on my face," says pro surfer Stephanie Gilmore. "It's healing. You can leave it on for five to ten minutes and you think it's super sticky, but it washes right off."

SCALP SCRUB

If the elements have left your scalp itchy or irritated, New York dermatologist Francesca Fusco, M.D., recommends this exfoliating concoction: add 1 teaspoon of salt or sugar to your regular shampoo and scrub away.

YOGURT AND TURMERIC MASK

Priyanka Chopra swears by this combination: "I'll put on fresh yogurt as a mask with a little turmeric powder in it—this is like an Indian trick," she says, particularly calling the spice "a healer for your skin."

FINISHING RINSE

According to colorist Christophe Robin, this hair rinse does wonders for keeping greasy roots at bay. Combine 1 part apple cider vinegar to 3 parts cold water and douse on scalp after shampooing and conditioning.

SUGAR LIP SCRUB

"My summer lip chap situation can be a little extreme, and I have a homemade trick to moisturize on the plane," says Gabrielle Union-Wade. "I figured out how to make a home scrub with brown sugar and olive oil, and I use that to exfoliate my lips. I keep a little container of it in my purse."

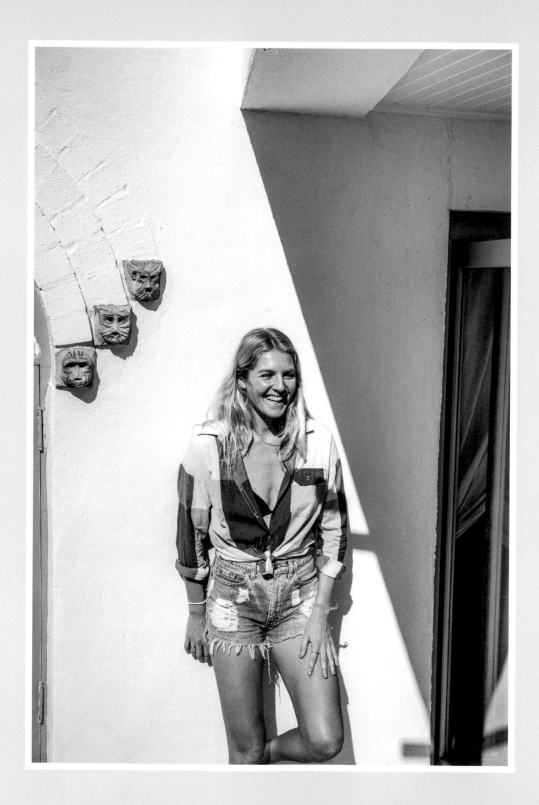

Stephanie Gilmore

Surfer

SKIN CARE

I'm in and out of the ocean; I'm constantly in the elements. So the whole basis of my skin care is getting enough moisture and, obviously, protection from the sun. In the morning, I don't really do much. I'll wake up and head straight to the surf. I use a sunscreen called Shade—I just found it about a year ago, and I've tried every sunscreen on the planet. It's a tinted SPF and it's all natural. It's perfect for the surf because it kind of sits on your face, but you don't look crazy putting it on because of the tint. That's a big thing for me because often in competitions, I'm coming in from a heat and then have to go on camera straightaway. And I have five of the Blistex SPF 20 DCT lip balm pots—one in each bag so I am never without.

If my lips are extremely chapped, I use pure vitamin E oil in a squeeze bottle. Or if I ever get a sunburn, I'll put honey on my face. It's healing. You can leave it on for five to ten minutes and you think it's super sticky, but it washes right off. It's a beautiful little trick of mine.

When I come in, I'll take the sunscreen off. If you have a good sunscreen, it'll be difficult to get off. I use the Derma E Makeup Remover— you can get it at Whole Foods. It does the job without completely ripping your skin off. Then I use a cleanser, an Australian product from

MooGoo, that feels creamy going on. I also use the brand's moisturizer. I think the brand originated from farms—the cream was used to repair cow udders. Sometimes at night, I'll add on this Obagi vitamin C serum. My sister actually got it first from a dermatologist and she told me to try it out. It improves my pigmentation. Obviously, if I'm traveling, I don't have access to everything, so I'll use the Clarins Beauty Flash Balm. It's super easy to use and soaks right in.

HAIR

I've never dyed my hair. It's really blonde and it's got a natural beach-y texture—basically from what the saltwater and sun does to it. But it also sucks up whatever moisture I put into it in three seconds. I can't live without my It's a 10 Miracle Leave-in Product. I spray it on after I surf or after a shower. Pretty much every girl on the professional surfing tour has it.

For shampoo, I'll use Evo—it's another Aussie brand. I really like a lot of the Australian products; they're doing a good job of using natural ingredients. Conditioner, I just go for Pantene. There's something about Pantene that coats your hair. I feel like it sort of protects your hair in the surf. And once every two weeks, I do a Kérastase hydrating mask.

For haircuts, one of the surfers on tour, Fred Patacchia, his wife, Missy, is a beautician by trade and she ends up cutting my hair. It's cool because she understands the surf and the elements and she keeps it pretty simple.

MAKEUP

My eyebrows and eyelashes get super light in the sun. So I like to get my lashes tinted every three to four weeks. If I'm out of the water, I'll add some Givenchy mascara. I prefer to draw my eyebrows in with this Bobbi Brown eyebrow kit, that way I have the option of wearing them light or dark.

I use the MAC Studio Face and Body Foundation. One of my good friends, who is a model in Australia, got me on all these MAC products. I also use the MAC Prep + Prime, but I use it for contour. Also, Rae Morris brushes have changed the way I work with makeup—they make everything go on natural. I'm always trying for that dewy, bronzed beach-babe look—it was all about Elle Macpherson when I was growing up and now I'm really obsessed with Gigi Hadid.

At night, I might do a Chanel cream foundation compact, which is a little thicker. I'm also loving these little MAC Paint Pots—I've been using the Groundwork color—that you can put on with just one finger swipe across the eye. Then, I'll do a little cat eye—I only do half the lid and not the bottom—with a L'Oréal liner. And I love the Chanel Rouge Coco Lipshines because they aren't too dry. For day, I use Interlude and at night I've been going a little more "French aggressive," which is how my Met Gala stylist referred to it, with Fiction.

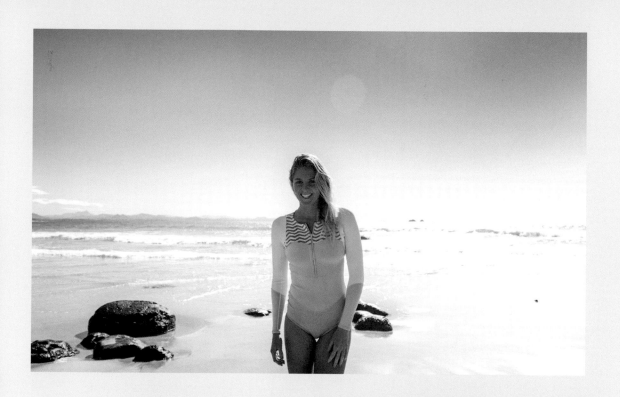

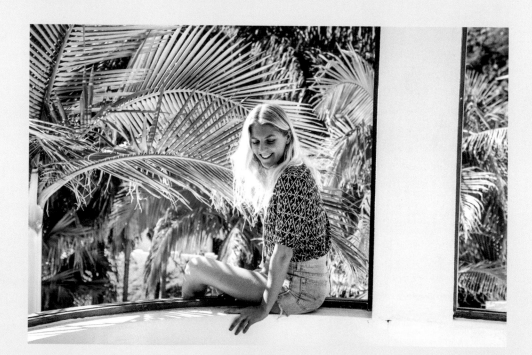

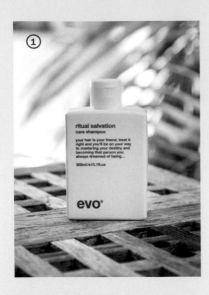

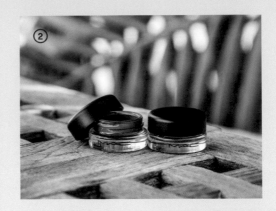

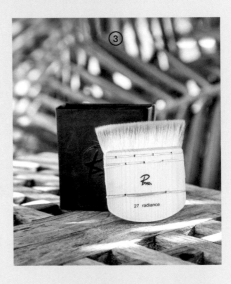

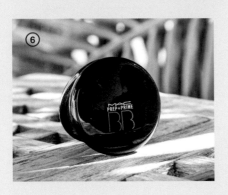

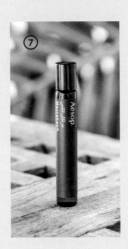

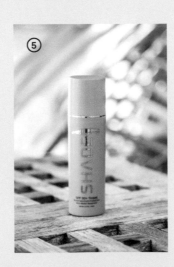

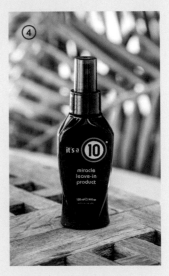

1 **Evo** Ritual Salvation
Shampoo

2 **MAC Paint Pots**
Groundwork

3 **Rae Morris** brush

4 **It's a 10** Miracle
Leave-in Product

5 **Shade**
Tinted SPF

6 **MAC** Prep + Prime
BB compact

7 **Aesop**
Marrakech Intense

FRAGRANCE

I've got three go-to fragrances. It kind of depends on what's going on and happening. For an evening out or something stronger, I like the Diptyque L'Ombre dans l'Eau. For everyday stuff, I've been using this little roll-on by Aesop called Marrakech Intense. The third scent—if I'm traveling, I don't want a crazy scent because nothing is worse than sitting next to someone on the plane doused in scent—is pure orange blossom oil that I got from a little fragrance shop in Byron Bay.

SERVICES

I know gels aren't that good for you, but it's the only thing that will stay on my nails. I love the fun and bright colors. At the moment, I have them in Barbie pink, which I guess goes with the whole Barbie girl beauty theme here!

On the world surfing tour, we have physiotherapists and chiropractors and masseuses at every destination we go to. We're pretty lucky there.

At home, I'm always seeing a chiropractor to make sure I'm straight. And I love to stretch.

DIET AND FITNESS

Surfing is pretty intense. It uses pretty much your entire body and it's pretty explosive. It's also very hard on your shoulders and knees and ankles. I'm always training to prevent injuries. I work with a guy, Nam Baldwin, and he'll mix it up. Lately, we've been doing martial arts stuff. It relates to surfing because it's about balance and core strength. You're trying to be in the most powerful stance you can be. We'll add in boxing and little courses where I have to jump over things. And we'll do stuff in the swimming pool called breath-hold: You get your heart rate up then dive under water and hold your breath as long as you can. It's a mental game and teaches you how to relax.

I have no real strict diet that I stick to, but I do keep it fresh. There's nothing better than a beautiful piece of fish with a yummy salad. But I've definitely got a sweet tooth. I have a Thermomix—it's a crazy machine that blends and cooks—and my specialty is orange and almond cake. You basically boil two whole oranges until they get really soft and then you put them in the Thermomix with their skin on and add almond meal. It's really easy and I'll make it when people are over. That's one of my favorite things: to have a dinner party with my friends.

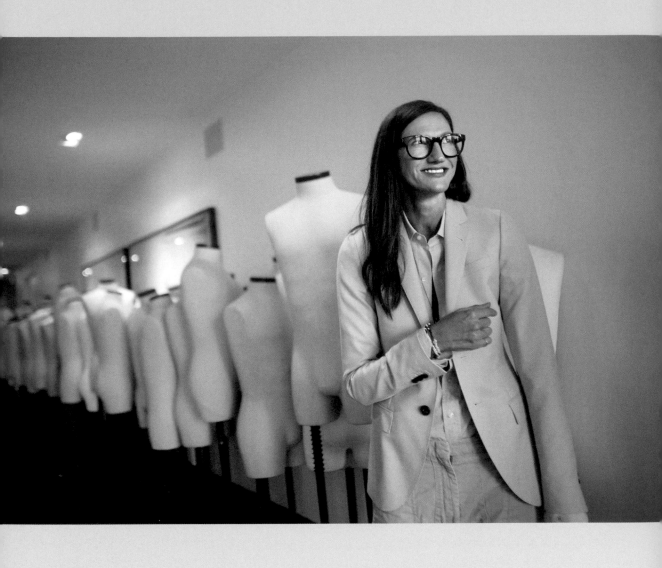

Jenna Lyons

Fashion Creative and Adviser

SKIN CARE

The woman I go to for facials, Aida Bicaj, recommended Biologique Recherche. That's how I start my day. I use the P50; it's my favorite thing that I don't leave home without. I have large ones, travel-size ones; I have them in the office, at home, in my pockets. Then, usually, I'll use an exfoliant by Arcona. They make a really fine scrub that I love.

I also have this Shiseido eye stuff I'm obsessed with. It's lightweight, and I'll put that all over my face, which is completely ridiculous. And I have this Shu Uemura big bottle of moisturizer and a small bottle of serum called Red: Juvenus Intense Vitalizing Concentrate. It comes with an eye dropper, which means it must

be good. There's also this Biologique Recherche bottle called Yall. It's not cheap. I only use it sometimes. I have to reserve my money for sofas and curtains and stuff. I'm hoping it makes me look younger, but I don't know. I just do what Aida tells me to do. I've been seeing her since I had my son. When he was born, I realized time was slipping away.

My nighttime routine starts with a glass of wine. I actually shower at night. I'm not a big fan of getting wet in the morning. I love Fresh Brown Sugar—just the name makes me happy—scrub and body wash. I wish I could say I consistently do the same skin care as in the morning, but I'd be lying. That's probably why I have so many wrinkles. It's the same stable of products though. Also, I am kind of obsessed with this Premium

Firming Sleeping Mask by Dr. Jart+. Sometimes I'll even use it during the day.

MAKEUP

I use this Shu Uemura eye makeup palette. It has all different shades of brown and some pale pink. I don't have any eyelashes, even though I do wear mascara. I try. I love the Chantecaille one because it's not heavy. I have like four lashes and it looks silly if you goop on thick mascara. Then I'll use the Tom Ford eyeliner. I love how it has two different sides. I have to wear liquid liner. Since I don't have any lashes, I don't have a holding line. Anything other than liquid liner makes me look like a bug. I also have this Shiseido gray eyebrow pencil. I've been buying it since the seventh grade. I was walking by the counter in the mall one day and the woman there took pity on me. She called me over and said, "I have to do something about your eyebrows." She drew in my eyebrows and changed my life. I wish I remembered her name; I should thank her!

For lips, I love the bright oranges and coral pinks from Bite Beauty. And I do wear foundation, but I haven't really found the perfect one. I need help with that. A lot of them go in my eyes.

For night, I actually change it up a lot. I love nothing more than a smoky eye, but then it's no lip. One of my favorites: a Bobbi Brown navy shadow that makes my eyes look light even though they are dark brown. The other thing I love is this pot of sparkly eye stuff by Stila. You mix it with a little drop of solution that comes with it and make this paste. It's total high school stuff.

FRAGRANCE

I'm pretty religious about perfume. I've been wearing Creed Silver Mountain Water for years. It's something that I want to hide because I don't want anyone to smell like me. The last year, I've been working with Arquiste on J. Crew scents, which has been such an interesting experience. I'd come home wearing the trial samples, and I noticed that scent changes the way people respond to you. For me, my scent has become part of my personality.

HAIR

I love Sachajuan shampoo and leave-in conditioner. A woman at work told me about it. I also use this Oribe moisturizing cream, which is incredible. I got a good sample at C. O. Bigelow and was hooked. This summer, I put it in my hair and would go into the salt water and get that beach-y look.

But I don't get my hair cut or dyed. I had a haircut disaster at forty. Actually, let me backtrack. At thirty, I cut bangs and everyone said it was the biggest mistake of my life. Then, for some reason, at forty, I took a picture of Alexa Chung and tried to get my hair cut like hers. I don't look like her; my hair texture is nothing like hers. Who knows why I did it! A friend from California was staying with me and her first reaction was, "Oh my god, I thought you were wearing a wig." I've been

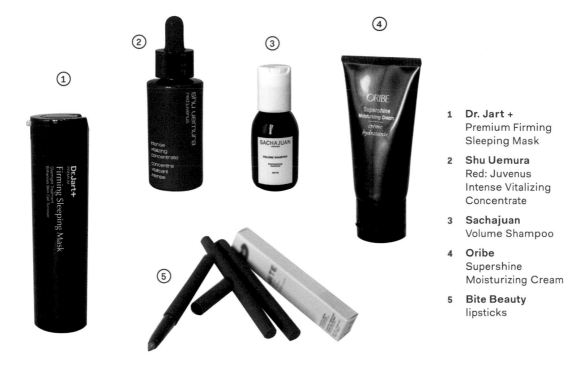

1 **Dr. Jart +**
Premium Firming
Sleeping Mask

2 **Shu Uemura**
Red: Juvenus
Intense Vitalizing
Concentrate

3 **Sachajuan**
Volume Shampoo

4 **Oribe**
Supershine
Moisturizing Cream

5 **Bite Beauty**
lipsticks

recovering from that haircut, which was years ago. I literally haven't had my hair cut since. But after having the kid, my hair stopped growing anyway. It also changed drastically in consistency. I don't even have words you can print to describe it: It's gotten thinner in some patches, coarser in others. It's completely irregular. Hence, the hairstyle: I always wear it slicked back so no one can tell what's going on. Things are going downhill, let me tell you. Oh well.

SERVICES

I try to see Aida every two to three months. For nails, honestly, I've gotten into the habit of doing them only for special occasions. Every once in a while, I'll have my nails done by Jin Soon [Choi]—she has her own nail polish line. About three months ago, I started getting massages by Nikki Yarnell; she'll come to the house. I'm becoming older and older by the minute and less mobile. The first time I called Nikki,

my hip and back were hurting, and I didn't have time to visit my favorite place in the whole wide world: the Greenwich Hotel spa. The pool there is incredible.

DIET AND FITNESS

I lift some really heavy sequins during the day. And I walk in five-inch heels regularly, which I believe is really good for my calves. Do we *have* to talk about diet and fitness?

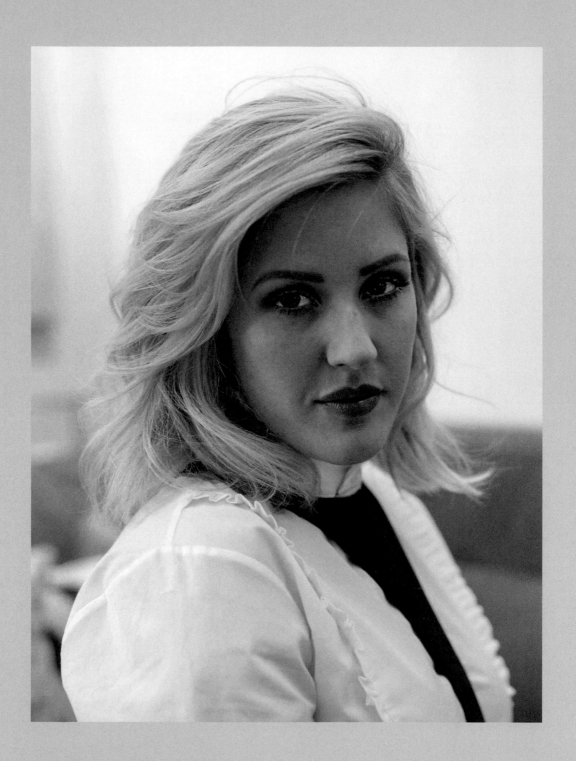

Ellie Goulding

Musician

MAKEUP

My makeup fascination is from watching my mom do it when I was growing up. She's really good at it. I tend to keep a pretty natural look and then I do dramatize it for the stage. So with MAC, they wanted to do a very specific collaboration in that the collection is basically made up of the colors I wear. I like the idea of a compact because it fits my lifestyle. You put it on in the morning and then you can take it with you. I've been using the Halcyon Days one. I fill in my brows with a Sisley Paris brow pencil—the line has really beautiful colors that are long lasting. And if I'm not using my MAC lipsticks or glosses, then I also love Charlotte Tilbury's lip color in Bitch Perfect, which is a pink-nude and stays on really well. I'm blonde and not dark so I tend to shy from a red lip.

I'll use mascara and I do love lots and lots of lashes. Before Lucy Wearing, my makeup artist, started coming on tour with me, I'd do my own makeup for stage and I'm quite good at lashes. Actually, we had a party for New Year's Eve and I did all my friends' lashes.

SKIN CARE

I usually shower in the morning and then I'll come out and use a toner. I tend to get quite glow-y skin and this toner by Pixi, which is vegan and animal friendly and is generally a brand I love, helps with that. And then I'll usually use a Rodial serum. I tend to go for a serum more than I do a moisturizer because I also use a very small amount of sunless tan. I love being tan and I don't like to use sun beds so I've become a self-tan expert. I like James Read, and the best one is the Express Glow Mask. The color develops very quickly so you don't somehow end up darker than you wanted to be in the middle of the day.

If I'm doing a shoot or performing, I particularly like a water-based makeup remover called Bioderma Sensibio H2O. When you're on a shoot and going through multiple looks, your eyes can get pretty sore with the makeup changes. This one is really gentle.

If I have time—I don't do it very often—I'm really into the Rodial Dragon's Blood Eye Masks. I've been obsessed with Rodial for a few years now, and they also have this Super Acids X-Treme Hangover Mask that is quite realistic I think. People may have a drink or two and then use this in the morning.

FRAGRANCE

I wear one by Christian Dior called Gris Montaigne. It's lovely but also unisex. I discovered it while literally walking in a department store. Someone working there sprayed me as I walked by. At first I was annoyed, but then it smelled quite nice. I can even spray on a couple spritzes and it's not overwhelming. Another one I like is Black Opium by YSL. It's so beautiful; I understand why it's a best-seller. That's one I'd wear in the evening.

HAIR

I'm desperately trying to get my hair to grow. I've always been a long hair kind of girl. When I look at pictures of myself, I always think I really want my long hair back. Also, you still need a good length of healthy hair to put extensions in. I'm not afraid of admitting I use extensions and spray tan. That's what I do and that's what a lot of girls do. I find it fun. Anyway, I had a hair disaster recently and I ended up having to cut my hair really short. Around the time I was promoting my album in New York, it was the best that my hair has been. Now it's kind of short because of the disaster and I've resisted the temptation of dying it—my roots are down to my ears! I've been using this product called F.A.S.T., which is supposed to make your hair grow fast, but I've been using it for a few weeks now and I haven't seen a difference. Otherwise, usually I use Kérastase volumizing shampoo and conditioner. You know when you find a shampoo that works for you? This is it.

For styling products, I'm very specific on what I use. I use BC Repair Rescue Sealed Ends by Schwarzkopf. I've dyed my hair and have had a lot of treatment. This is not really a cream and not really an oil, but it works. Then I'll use Oribe Maximista Thickening Spray. It smells so good and I love having my hair bigger and more dramatic, especially if I'm going out.

Because I'm often on the road, my hair is cut and dyed by people all over the board. If I'm in London, I'll get my extensions done at Easton Regal and I'll get my hair cut by Louis Byrne.

OTHER SERVICES

At Hershesons, I'll get a good body scrub in preparation for a tan. I'll also get my nails done

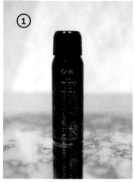

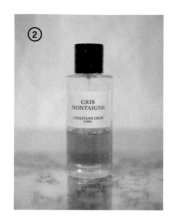

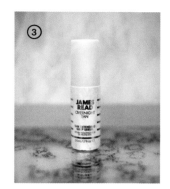

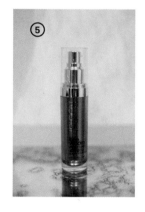

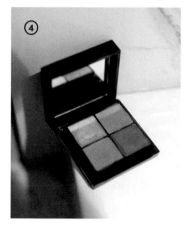

1 **Oribe**
Dry Texturizing Spray

2 **Christian Dior**
Gris Montaigne

3 **James Read**
Overnight Tan

4 **MAC Compact**
Ellie Goulding
Collection

5 **Rodial**
Bee Venom

there. I get Shellac because I don't have time to keep up with normal nail varnish.

DIET AND FITNESS

I like to run; I like to box; I like do Barry's Bootcamp. I like a mix of things. I just went to Norway for a few days and we were climbing mountains and dogsledding. Dogsledding was so good! At first it was really scary—they go so fast and it can be very messy if the sled overturns—but it was so incredible. It was minus 30° out and I stupidly only took my serum. My skin was kind of dry but it has since recovered.

I'm a vegetarian. I don't eat fish or meat. I also try my best to not have dairy or animal products. For breakfast, I had kale with rye bread and a green juice. But I'd say I'm generally pretty balanced. I do have vices like alcohol and chocolate. I'm not too hard on myself about sugar. I know many people who are into health and fitness who are antisugar and antigluten. But with my job being the way it is, I can't be too strict about things. If I'm doing a sound check and there is only a limited amount of food at the venue, I'll find something to eat.

Nina Dobrev

Actress

HAIR

My hair is a few inches below my shoulder right now. I've been dying to cut my hair for the last seven years: to cut it pretty short, but not like boy short. I did that in grade six and I looked like a boy. I actually had to wear dresses, otherwise I was mistaken for one. I wouldn't go that short again, but maybe an above-the-shoulder bob. But because I was on *Vampire Diaries* for so many years, contractually, I was not allowed.

I'm looking forward to having a role coming up so I can cut it. Riawna Capri, my hairstylist, is also dying to do it. I actually met her through a friend of mine who was getting his hair cut. As I was sitting in the chair in the salon, she was looking at me and she was like, "You need some help. Your hair looks dull and you need a little trim." She gave me a gloss treatment and she trimmed my hair and didn't even charge me. I had just moved to L.A. and I didn't even have a show. There was no reason to suck up to me in any way. I didn't see her for about a year after that. But when I had my first movie to promote, I had my agent reach out to her to do my hair. We've become really good friends since. We have the same energy. She's so positive.

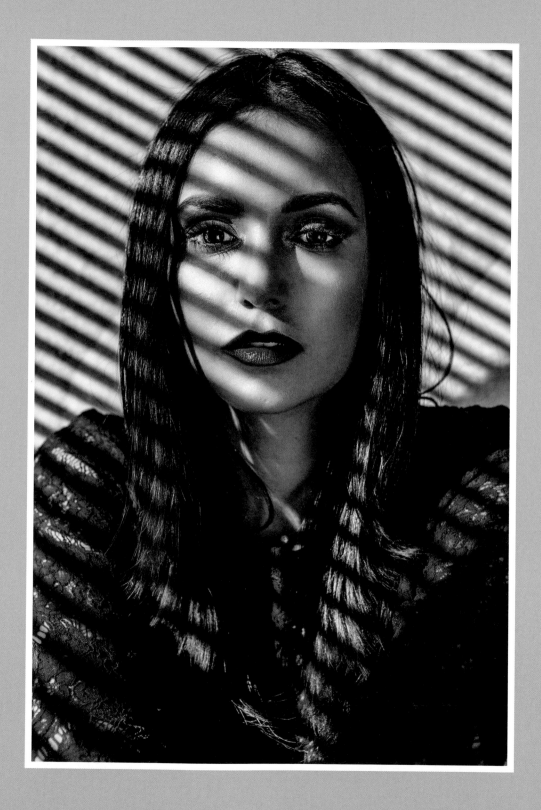

Anyway, right now, this is my natural color. I've had ombré in the past and a whole bunch of different things. I use a lot of Unite products because Riawna suggested them. They're amazing. They smell great and are incredibly moisturizing. There's one called 7SECONDS Detangler that you spray and leave in. I have naturally curly hair; I can walk out of the shower, use the spray, and I'll have beach-y, wavy hair. But otherwise I'm not especially good at doing my own hair; that's not my forte.

FRAGRANCE

I do like fragrance but minimally. I have two signature scents. They are Burberry Body for night, but day-to-day I use Fresh, the Hesperides Grapefruit spray. I don't overdo it. I like my natural pheromones to have a chance.

SKIN CARE

In the morning, I press my snooze button about fifteen to thirty times and then I go to my bathroom to splash cold, cold water on my face. I have a pretty specific regimen after that. I always wash with my cleanser by Kate Somerville and then Lancer The Method: Polish to exfoliate. But for the most part, I do all Kate Somerville. The way I found out about Kate is through Riawna. I do the Nourish Daily Moisturizer and I have the DermalQuench as well. I hydrate with that a couple times a day. I even have a travel-size one in my purse. I'm sort of obsessed with all things travel-size. They're so cute looking and adorable. But it's also because I'm on a plane every four to five days. I have to stay moisturized. I also use Kiehl's Creme de Corps on my body.

MAKEUP

When I'm not working, I don't really wear makeup. But I like to counteract that with a lip for that reason. I might do a strong lip color that will sort of create the illusion that there's stuff there. One of the items I love is the NARS Velvet Lip Glide. I have it in a brighter pinkish-red; I like bold colors.

But if I am wearing foundation—everyone has a blemish or dark circles from lack of sleep at some point—my go-to is Chanel Perfection Lumière Velvet. It covers well but not too much. Also, it has powder built into the foundation. It's great for someone on the go.

I might do a little bit of contouring. I was taught by a makeup artist. There are certain parts of your face you should accent: the cheekbones, the bridge of your nose, and above your eyebrows. I use different bronzers depending on my mood, but I do prefer matte ones. I always try to go more natural. You get enough sparkle from the sunshine in L.A.

I love Kevyn Aucoin for eyeshadows. The colors are more matte and I have an earth-tone palette. My complexion is more bronze-y and dark so it works. For mascara, I love Benefit They're Real! For eyeliner, I go back and forth between a liquid one by Dior and one by an Asian brand that I discovered when

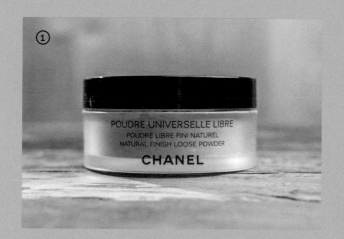

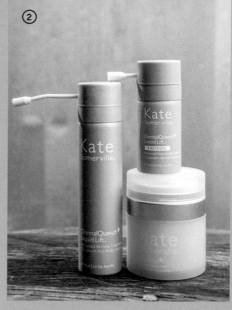

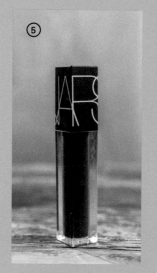

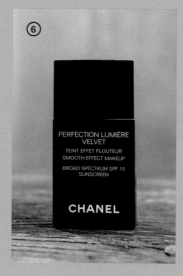

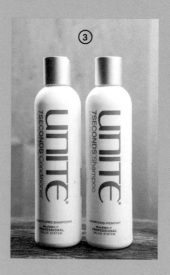

1 **Chanel**
Natural Finish Loose
Powder

2 **Kate Somerville**
DermalQuench
Liquid Lift products

3 **Unite** 7SECONDS
Shampoo,
Conditioner

4 **Kiehl's**
Creme de Corps

5 **NARS**
Velvet Lip Glide

6 **Chanel**
Perfection Lumière
Velvet

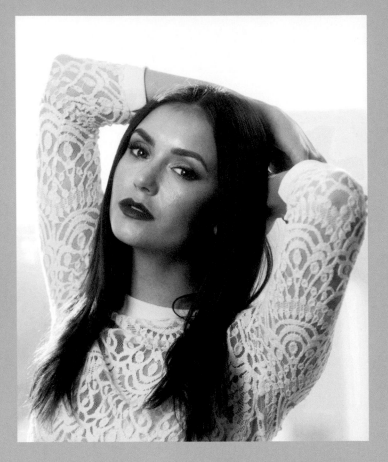
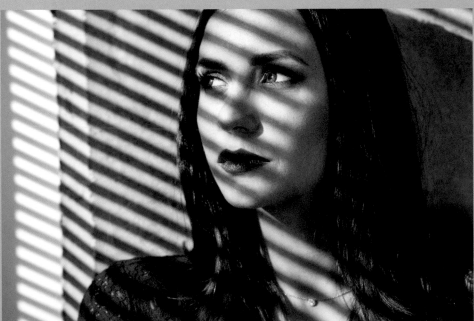

I was traveling for press. They're doing something right in Asia; it does not budge. If I'm going out, I love a cat eye. Audrey Hepburn is a big inspiration for me, and her look was a lot of cat eye.

OTHER SERVICES

I am obsessed with acupuncture and massage. I get a lot of massages, perhaps an unhealthy amount. I'll probably get them once a week or maybe once every two weeks. It's a very bougie habit to have. There's a place called The NOW in L.A. It's very low-key and chill and doesn't feel like you're in a massage mill even though that's all they do there.

DIET AND FITNESS

I've always been health conscious and very active. I grew up in a household with boys and loved sports. But as an adult, I still try to do things that are fun. It's more fun to do something that doesn't feel like a workout. But recently, I was on a movie and they hired a trainer for me. For the first time, I was working out with weights in a gym and I was so afraid to bulk up, but I discovered it all depends on how you work out with them. Now I've been keeping it up. I've been working out with Harley Pasternak.

I try to stay away from pastas as much as I love them, but I do cheat a lot. You have to live a happy life and not restrict yourself too much. I just work out a little harder. You do have pressures in this industry. Your appearance is part of your job. But beauty is not just a superficial thing. I really think it's very multifaceted and multilayered and goes from the inside out. It's important to keep your brain stimulated and your insides, what you put in your body, healthy. If you have a happy heart and you have a happy face, then that's probably the most beautiful thing to me.

RACHEL GOODWIN
ON CAMERA-READY SKIN THAT LOOKS BEAUTIFUL IN REAL LIFE

When you're working inches away from your client's face for hours at a time, energy matters. That's one main reason I reach out to L.A.-based Rachel Goodwin for beauty advice. (I'm not the only one: She tends to Emma Stone and Brie Larson before major appearances.) She's mellow, down for a laugh but also quite the perfectionist—especially when it comes to skin matters. Her meticulous yet natural-looking foundation application is something to behold.

Right now, there are a couple schools of thought on camera-ready skin. The approach is very divided at the moment. Let me backtrack. For me, the dawn of the HD cameras was really when I started to understand skin. Up to that point, makeup artists approached makeup as how to trick the camera. How do we get this makeup on to trick the lighting or in a way that uses the lighting? This idea came from film make-up in the early 1920s and '30s. At that time, if a woman had an eye that was slightly smaller—and no one has perfectly symmetrical features—you would do corrective makeup to fix that. You could get away with different types of things back then because the camera wasn't exactly telling the truth. Lighting could be used to create shadows and dimension.

Pancake makeup was invented for that specific thing. Pancake has been around for a long time. But then in the '80s and '90s, the foundation formulas started changing. There was a Kevyn Aucoin stage and the music-video era, which influenced what people wanted: less stuff on the skin. Then with HD, the formulas changed again. Now there are two camps:

1. The social media artists who have popularized doing these intense beauty looks with matte lips and tons of contouring. This is coming straight from the '20s and '30s. Is there a place for it? Clearly. There are tons of women who are into it. That style of makeup, to me though, looks incredibly dated. It comes down to an aesthetic choice.

2. My approach is this: If my client is going to the Oscars and she is going to be on camera, I know she is going to be in front of people as well. I don't want her to look like a caricature. I want her to look beautiful, but it also better look good with a camera right up in her face. My approach is that skin is the most important thing. It's about creating that translucency, that realness, that lushness, that vitality. I don't like the way makup looks when it's covering up the skin—rather, skin needs to look alive and she, my client, needs to be the best version of herself.

HOW TO GET BELIEVABLE CAMERA-READY SKIN

I start with a full-coverage foundation, but I use it very lightly. I want the most amount of coverage with the least amount of product.

I like to use a beautyblender and spritz rose water on it. Then I sponge on the makeup. When you press it on, it leaves just a slight trace of foundation. In fact, when you're doing this stippling motion, you're actually applying the product and removing it at the same time.

Use a high-coverage foundation very strategically. Just use it where it's needed. Maybe you'll use it around the nose, for blemishes, and under the eyes. Leave the rest of the skin as nude or translucent as possible.

A highlighter can be effective for creating that "living skin" look. I love the RMS Living Luminizer for that. But just a touch: You don't want to end up looking robotic. My approach here is less is more.

There's a place for powder, especially on the red carpet. If it's a hot day and my client is going to be there for hours, I tend to use a loose, really sheer powder and then only on the center of the face, middle of the forehead, and edges of the lip.

If you have particularly oily skin, don't pile on the powder. Instead, there are these incredible living matte foundations now. They're really a breakthrough. They give a wonderful finish without looking like those '90s mattes that we all remember. Somehow, with these new formulas, the skin still comes through. I use them often on press junket days when I don't want to powder the girl twenty times a day.

On primers: They can be incredible when someone has really textured skin. Bobbi Brown makes a good one. But I don't think they're necessary for every day. The truth is, primers don't really help things stay on. I get that brands are selling makeup and kind of need to tell that story, but it actually ends up going the other way. If you're layering and layering product (which is against my philosophy in general), that's just more stuff that can come off. More products on the skin are just more products on the skin.

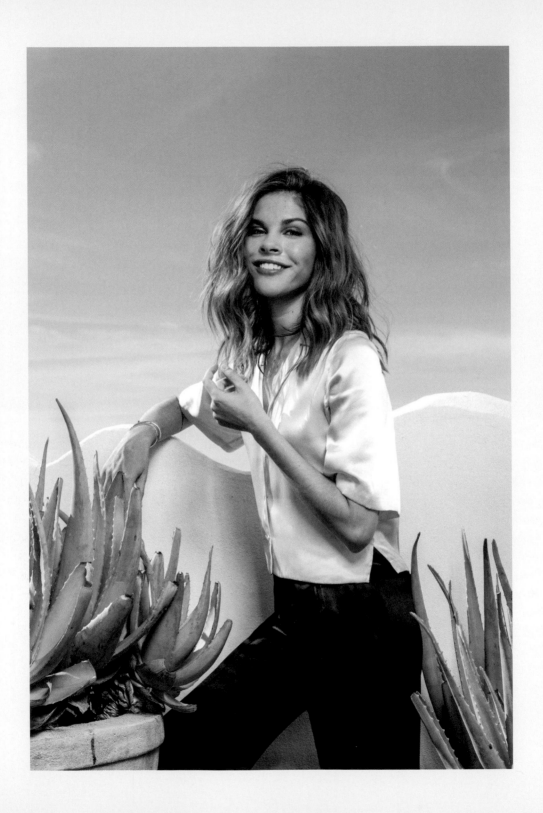

Emily Weiss

Founder of the Beauty Brand

Glossier

SKIN CARE

I've had an interesting journey from beauty editor to beauty product creator. Part of being a beauty product creator now is trying a million and one different submissions of stuff. We narrow down what we're going to make anywhere from six months to a year out, and then we're in the process of trying on submissions. We can have anything from thirty to forty different serums for one product. Every morning, I have a new bag from our product development team with a little note saying, "Here's what you need to try." Every morning, I have beauty homework. But there are some things that are tried and true that I use every day.

Cleanser-wise, I use the Tracie Martyn Amla Purifying Cleanser, which I actually have used for, like, five years. As a beauty editor, there are so few products you actually keep using. This one is great because it gently brightens and clarifies. I think it has some sort of alpha hydroxy situation and some organic, natural enzymes. At night, I'll use Milky Jelly Cleanser from Glossier, because it takes off mascara and makeup really, really well.

My day-to-day moisturizer has always been the Priming Moisturizer by Glossier. Before the moisturizer, I'll layer in actives like serums. There's one called Good Genes by Sunday Riley that also has a gentle exfoliating action, although lately it's been making my skin feel a little tight. Then there are the Supers, our serums. If I know I'm doing makeup, I'll use the Super Bounce one— it makes my skin cushion-y and plumped up.

Eye creams—I've never found one I loved so much that I stuck with it. There's a Clinique one that I use. And there are samples I got from Aida Bicaj that are from Valmont.

I used the P50 from Biologique Recherche when I was getting a lot of hormonal acne on my chin-strap area. It really cleared it up and I never got it again. Now I use it occasionally, maybe once every two weeks when I need a deep clean. The thing about P50 is that after you use it, your face is fire-engine red—like a burn victim—but it works. There's also a retinol product from Shani Darden. I think it's working and there are no negative side effects. For me, it's all about skin.

MAKEUP

Most days—I would say five days out of the week—I don't use any makeup. None today. Literally, I slept from midnight to three last night. I guess that's when you're supposed to use makeup, but I'm like screw it.

When I do want to put in the effort, I do the same thing every time. I do the Perfecting Skin Tint in Medium when my moisturizer is still drying.

It's sort of like a filter for your face, but it's not pancake face. Then I do Stretch Concealer in Medium, which I use more like finger paint. I put it under my eyes and around my nose and under my lips. I use a Smashbox blush called Silver Lake Sunset. It's a cream blush stick. Actually, I do, like, a three-part cheek thing. I do the blush, which is like a less sparkly NARS Orgasm, on my proper cheek. Then I layer the matte NARS bronzing stick under my cheekbones for a little shadow and pull it down because the makeup artist Wendy Rowe said it's what she does on Kate Moss and she calls it "cool girl blush." Then, for a highlight on my brow bone and under my eyes, I use our Haloscope in Quartz, which is a dewy effect. I do Kevyn Aucoin mascara—it's the one with the tiny brush. I hate when there's too much product on a mascara brush. I almost prefer when it's dried out. This one also has tubing and I love the fact that it just slides off when you want it to.

I'll use RMS Eye Polish in Solar really close to the lash line. It's a really perfect gold. I do Glossier Boy Brow in Brown. Then I'll use a loose powder just from anywhere and I'll dust some powder on my T-zone so I'm not too shiny. Also, I use our Balm Dotcom every day. That's my classic lip balm that I put on my lips after the shower.

My favorite lipstick, when I do wear it, is Cake from Glossier. I wore it on the day of my wedding. Otherwise, I don't really wear anything on my lips.

HAIR

I've had many a hair journey. I'm thirty-one: I've been platinum, I've had a mullet, I've had a Leonardo DiCaprio circa the '90s haircut. My best look is just shoulder length.

One thing that has always worked on my hair, though, is Christophe Robin Cleansing Purifying Scrub with Sea Salt. It's a great product because my hair is very straight and it's very fine, but I have a lot of it. Anything I can use to beef it up that's not a styling agent, I'm for. I don't love styling product. But

①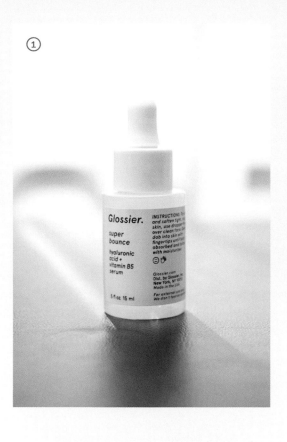

②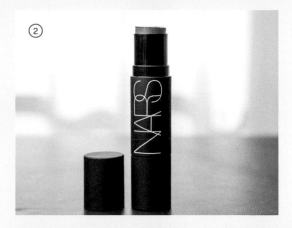

③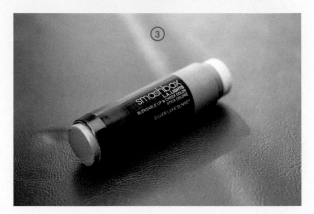

1	**Glossier**	4	**Sunday Riley**
	Super Bounce		Good Genes
			Treatment
2	**NARS**		
	bronzing stick	5	**Kevyn Aucoin**
			The Volume
3	**Smashbox**		Mascara
	L.A. Lights		

④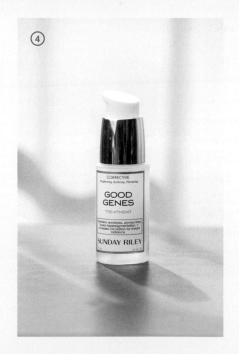

⑤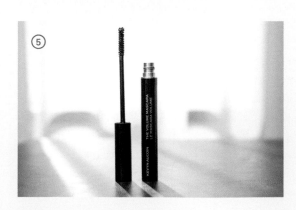

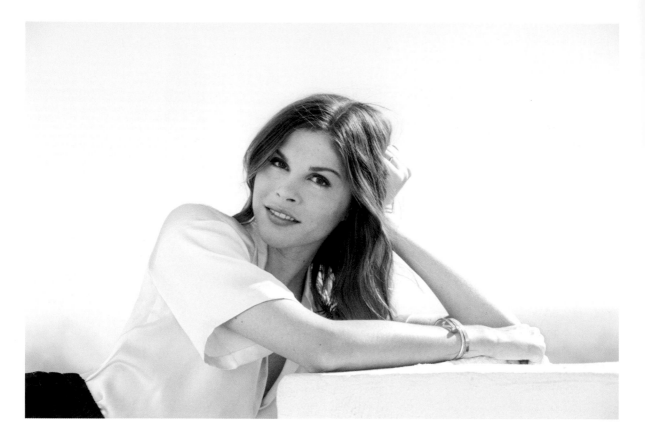

I find this gives it a little grit. It gives it more of that French, beefed-up kind of texture.

I got some highlights in Copenhagen from Mia, who works at Studio Cim Mahony. I've gone twice to Copenhagen but not just for hair! But when I'm there to visit friends, I'll schedule the highlights. So, I use the Christophe Robin Shade Variation Care Nutritive Mask in Ash Brown or Purple. It keeps the tone from going in the wrong direction.

I guess for styling product, I do like the Aveda dry shampoo. You turn the nozzle and it sprinkles—it's not an aerosol. That Shampure smell is just so good. If I'm doing a side-part sleek pony, I'll use Redken shine spray. It will smooth everything, and it does give you a high shine.

FRAGRANCE

I tend to latch onto a perfume for like one year and I wear it every day and I'm obsessed with it and then one day I wake up and I'm like, "Ugh, I can't wear this anymore." So I basically have a library of perfumes on my bathroom counter even though I don't wear some of them anymore because I'm on to the next one. There are some similar themes: I really like fragrances from Le Labo. I really enjoy fragrances from Byredo. I love both those founders as people. They're so creative and so clever. Right now, I really like the Le Labo L.A. fragrance Musc 25. I also like the one they did for Japan. They're both subtle, creamy whitewood scents. I also like

Kiehl's Musk and the other one I really like is Bonpoint's baby perfume. I'll do that sometimes at night when I get out of a really thorough shower. I'll just be like an extra-clean baby.

OTHER SERVICES

Sometimes, I'll use ZIIP; it's this microcurrent device by this aesthetician in L.A. called Melanie Simon. I got it for free—she sent it to me—and it syncs to an app on your phone, which tells you what to do. I think I've seen a difference. She tells you to do it twice a week. I don't think that's enough, because it only lasts about a day. There was a period of time for two weeks where I used it almost every day and I looked really good. If only I had the discipline.

I used to go, and I would still go if I had something special to get ready for, to Shamara Bondaroff of SB Skin. She's in Union Square and she's very holistic. She does proper microcurrents, probably 5,000x the power of my at-home device. I did it

before my wedding. But that's really time intensive and you basically have to do it three times a week. If I were Kim Kardashian, that would be fine for me, because that would be my job: to look really good. But I'm just in an office.

The other person I have to give huge credit to, and she's the best facialist I've ever been to in my life, is Isabelle Bellis. She's on the Upper East Side. Literally, you cannot get an appointment for a full year, because it's just her. She's magical. She's about homeopathic pure elements. Plus, she massages the inside of your mouth with a glove. She's very expensive, but it's a two-hour facial, so it's a big deal. I went for my wedding.

I also love getting a massage, but I'm inconsistent with who I go to. Every week, I'll just go to my corner nail place and get a chair massage.

Also, Lisa at Iris Nails at University and 10th Street does great nails. I'm overdue to see her. She was on vacation for like six weeks in August. My nails are a mess.

DIET AND FITNESS

I'm inconsistent with fitness. One workout that has worked for over a year, though, is Physique 57. It's a barre method class. I like strength resistance and things that make you long and lean. That's the dream for me. I'll go once a week on Sunday. I don't have a private trainer or anything. I just take a class.

Diet-wise, I just try to do everything in moderation. By that, I mean I'll have a green juice in the morning and a cookie by 3 P.M. From time to time, I'll do a cleanse. I like the principles of the Clean program by Dr. Alejandro Junger. His book is actually really good and you can do it yourself. And in this day and age, with all the crazy fad diets like Atkins, his book makes a lot of sense. Anything too extreme, maybe it's good in the short run, but what's that doing to you over time?

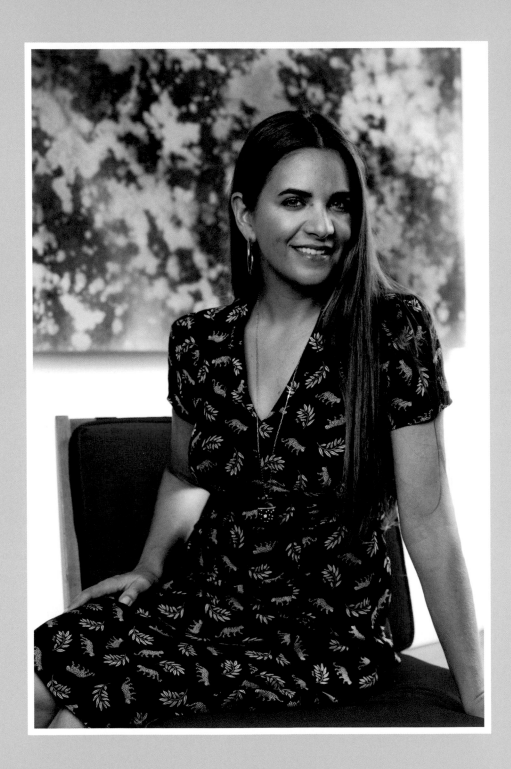

Laure Heriard Dubreuil

Cofounder of The Webster retail store

FRAGRANCE

Scent has always been something that's been very important to me. Even when I was five years old, I would remember the smell of my grandmother's perfume. I wanted to be a nose growing up. I developed the scent of The Webster, which is based on orange blossom. For me, Frédéric Malle scents are very special. I change between Lys Mediteranee and Dans tes Bras. I love also Portrait of a Lady. It depends on my mood and the time of day.

SKIN CARE

First thing I do, I use Sisley Paris Gel Nettoyant Gommant, which is the Buff and Wash Facial Gel. With that, I can exfoliate at the same time as I wash. And I can do it daily and it's not too harsh and gives you a glow. With my skin care and everything else, I'm really focusing on efficiency.

Once I find something is really working for me, I'm extremely faithful and I keep it. I don't have much time to try new things. For example, in the shower after I wash, use the Clarins body oils. I started using them when I was pregnant and I kept using them. The smell is amazing. You feel like you're in the spa but it takes just three minutes. It's efficient!

For my face, I'll put the Tata Harper serum on. Especially after the summer, my skin is a little bit dry. After that, and I've done this for the longest time, I use the Embryolisse Lait-Crème Concentrè. This is so good. I can use it for everything. I can use it on my son. I can use it even after a flight to hydrate. I have it in my handbag.

I wear sunscreen every day. I like the one from La Roche-Posay that's like a film you put on top of your day cream. It's not greasy. At night, I'll use the make-up removing Micelle Solution from Bioderma—the one with the pink cap—to take off makeup. Then, I put on the Embryolisse.

MAKEUP

Especially after the summer, if I still have the glow, I don't put on much foundation. But when I start to lose my glow, I use NARS Pure Radiant Tinted Moisturizer with SPF 30 on top of my cream. Then I just use mascara. I love the Yves Saint Laurent Effet Faux Cils. You don't need much. It makes a big impact when you're tired, especially when you have a two-year-old son!

Since I had my son, everything is on the go: makeup on the go, cream on the go, hair drying on the go. Just stick your head out the window of the car, ha!

The other thing that is wonderful is I use the Glossier Balm Dotcom. I put it everywhere I need a little glow, like my lips, maybe cheeks and eyelids.

For a party or an event, something I add is the Charlotte Tilbury Magic Cream. This really is magical if you're getting ready for an event. I put this on and I'm already a new person. I don't even need makeup anymore! During fashion week, I use the cream a lot because the rhythm is very intense.

I don't wear a lot of lipstick or lip color, but I recently discovered the Pat McGrath Labs lipsticks. They are matte and last a very long time and I have to say I love all those burgundy colors. I got one called Vermillion Venom, which is really incredible. It's like a red-aubergine. It comes in a whole kit with gloss and matching glitter. I have tried the glitter, but I haven't worn it out of the house yet. It's going to be my Paris Fashion Week thing or even for Halloween.

HAIR

I really love Leonor Greyl's palm oil. My hair is dry. This is great and nourishing. I also use it in the summer to protect from saltwater and chlorine. In the winter, I use it as a mask. I also use the Leonor Greyl shampoo and conditioner. But this summer when I was in Saint Tropez, I ran out and went to the pharmacy and tried the shampoo with dates from Klorane. I love the smell. I became addicted to it. You really feel like you're somewhere in Morocco and someone is making you this concoction of dates.

OTHER SERVICES

I do get massages a lot. I have an amazing woman who comes to the house. I found her through friends. I'd rather keep her name secret. She's going to become too busy! In New York, you can have anyone come to your house day or night. In Paris, so many things are closed early and you have to book far in advance. It's great for a working life to have this.

DIET AND FITNESS

I do yoga. I started when I was pregnant with my son and really loved it. Actually, my husband started doing it with me then and we've continued. When we travel, we have applications that we can use and it's quite easy to maintain it. But when we're in NYC, I go to Yoga to the People. It's right around the corner from our house.

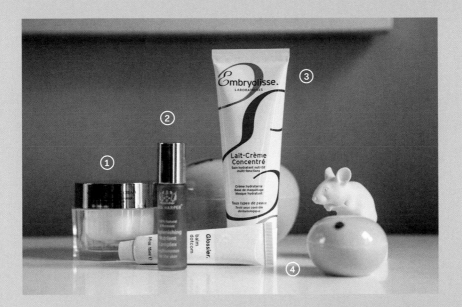

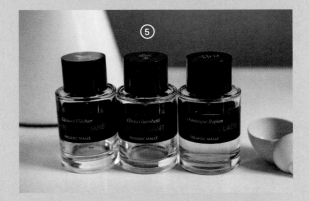

1. **Charlotte Tilbury**
   Magic Cream
2. **Tata Harper**
   Replenishing Nutrient
   Complex
3. **Embryolisse**
   Lait-Crème
   Concentré
4. **Glossier**
   Balm Dotcom
5. **Frédéric Malle**
   Lys Mediteranee,
   En Passant,
   Portrait of a Lady
6. **Sisley Paris**
   Gel Nettoyant
   Gommant
7. **Clarins**
   Body Treatment Oil
8. **Pat McGrath Labs**
   Vermillion Venom

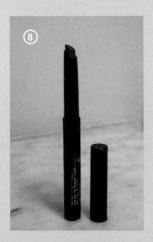

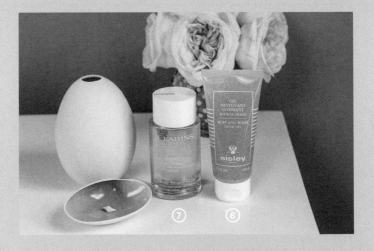

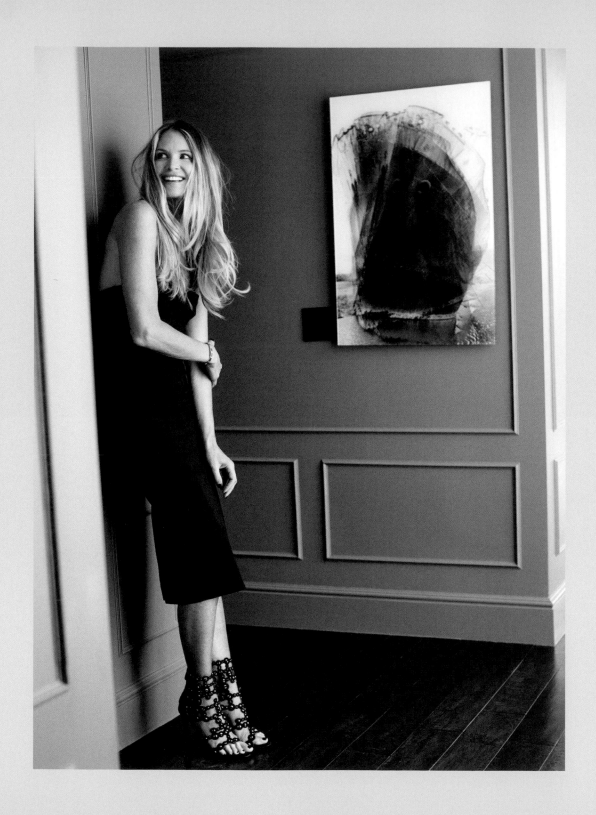

Elle Macpherson

Model and Entrepreneur

SKIN CARE

The first thing: I believe in beauty from the inside out. What you put in your body is more important than what you put on your body, although they do work in tandem.

Second thing is: I believe in exfoliation. The skin is the number one detox organ, so if I can exfoliate and get my circulation going, that's really important as well. I use a sea-salt scrub for my body twice a day. For my face, I'll use a glycolic wash cleanser by NeoStrata every day. Then a couple days a week, I'll also use a scrub or deeper exfoliator. I like the Dr. Sebagh one, which is acid-based and it's gentle. Or I'll use a Dr. Brandt one, which is like a face polish.

At the moment, I'm really loving the Crème de La Mer. It's rich and my skin has a tendency to get dehydrated from plane travel. Being based in Miami, sunblock is my number one friend. I like Invisible Zinc. I also like one by Dr. Brandt. For most of my products, I'll get recommendations from dermatologists or makeup artists. I like hearing about things word of mouth because there is so much product out there now and they all come in such beautiful packaging and they all promise the world. I get it confused, so that's why word of mouth is key. Like the eye cream I use is by Arianna Skincare. The way I heard about it was actually from Norman Foster's wife. Her skin looks amazing and I asked what she used. She suggested this eye cream, so I looked it up and it really works. I also like the Natura Bisse Diamond Life Infusion Retinol Eye Serum. Then for my lips and cuticles, I use Lucas' Papaw—it's very Aussie.

MAKEUP

I like a very natural face. I don't really wear any foundation at all. For every day, I use RMS Beauty products. They're coconut oil–based and they sit on the skin beautifully. I have one pot for the eyes and one pot for cheeks and lips. I do wear mascara: I like Diorshow Black Out. And I like a very, very pale brow. I do fill them in with the Bobbi Brown pencil in Ash, but I don't like it when the brow is dark. Everybody now is doing these exaggerated brows and it's not my thing. I like a strong frame as in the shape but I like the color to be very soft.

For a night out, I'll do a dark smoky eye. I'll use Bobbi Brown pencils then smudge. Then I'll do a lot of mascara and a pale lip. It has to be super simple—I'm not somebody who will spend an hour on makeup. I'm lucky if I'll spend ten minutes, even when I'm going out. Also, concentrating for hours on your face, I don't think it's healthy anyway. Living in Miami, it's obviously humid. There's a tendency to glow, but I like that. If I'm doing TV, I'll use MAC Studio Fix on my T-zone and it's really great for photography, TV, and film, but it's too much for every day. Chanel also has a great loose powder that I'll pop on my T-zone—it's more natural looking.

HAIR

For me, my hair is as important as my face. I've worked with Oribe for twenty to thirty years. He's still one of the best in the business, and when he came out with his own products, they were just superior to anything out there. I use his shampoos and conditioners. He's also based in Miami and we do see each other, but he's always so busy shooting.

I go to Josh Wood in London for my color. He keeps my hair looking modern, relevant, and natural. He doesn't just do a single process. He's encouraged me to use my natural roots. He does a sun-kissed look on the ends sometimes but he keeps the color looking strong and natural.

FRAGRANCE

I've worn Vetiver by Guerlain—it's a men's cologne—for maybe thirty years now. I smelled it on somebody once and then I wanted it for myself. But I'd like to create my own perfume. It's definitely in the cards.

SERVICES

I really believe in the fusion of Eastern and Western medicines. I do acupuncture and kinesiology—it's a form of body diagnosis through response of the body. I also do osteopathy. Massage is important to me, not just for relaxation but also for circulation. Nichola Joss does amazing facial and body massages.

DIET AND FITNESS

About three years ago, I started doing an alkaline diet.

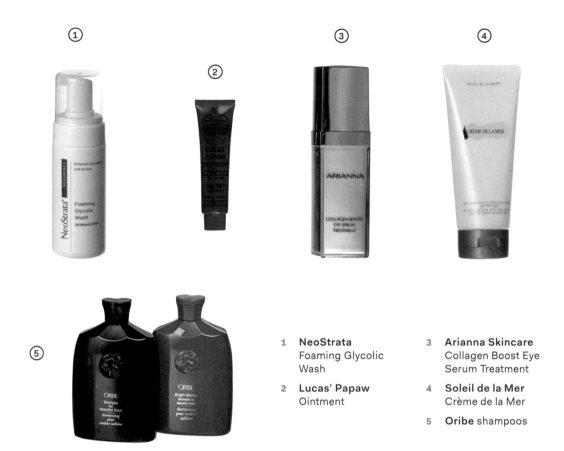

1 **NeoStrata**
Foaming Glycolic
Wash

2 **Lucas' Papaw**
Ointment

3 **Arianna Skincare**
Collagen Boost Eye
Serum Treatment

4 **Soleil de la Mer**
Crème de la Mer

5 **Oribe** shampoos

I was feeling listless and tired and lacked muscle tone. What I was doing before wasn't working as well. I went to a nutritionist and she did some testing and said I was too acidic. I did some minor changes to my diet, like less red meat, and she also gave me this green powder to drink. That's where the idea of my Super Elixir came from. I worked with that nutritionist and I put everything that I needed or wanted out of vitamins and supplements into one product.

I don't even consider doing fitness for fitness's sake. I like to be outdoors, and the way I choose to engage with the outdoors is through sport. In NYC, I'll run around the Reservoir. In Miami, I'll paddleboard or jet ski or run along the beach. If I'm in the mountains, I ski or hike. I like to play tennis even though I'm not very good at it. For me, it's more about the sport—it's not about needing to get a workout in or losing weight. I don't spend time at a gym. I don't have a trainer. But I do have friends who I love to do these activities with.

PATRICK TA
HOW TO
PERFECT MODERN
SMOKY EYES

I am interested in Patrick Ta for what he heralds: a power shift in the makeup artist world. In the past, an up-and-comer needed to earn his stripes by assisting other makeup artists. Instead, Los Angeles–based Ta circumvented the usual route by building his portfolio via Instagram. Certainly one look at his social media account and you'd see the young gun—he's still in his mid-twenties—is doing well for himself. Yes, there's the numbers game—he has plenty of followers—but also he's built credibility among the millennial set through who he works with: names like Gigi Hadid, Jenna Dewan Tatum, Olivia Munn, and Shay Mitchell. I can't help but admire his entrepreneurial spirit—isn't the modern way of beauty that rules are meant to be broken?—and also his playful use of color. A smoky eye doesn't have to read gray, black, and monotone shades in between. Ta, naturally, uses his own approach.

I didn't assist other makeup artists like many in my industry. Instead, I learned by working at a MAC Cosmetics counter, and I also learned through watching YouTube and studying pictures. Perhaps that's not the route many in my profession take, but at the counter, I was seeing just everyday people and doing makeup that was truly wearable. Being able to practice on so many different face types and skin tones has helped me tremendously in what I do now. Working at a counter also teaches you how to apply makeup very quickly. People are shopping; they have places to be. I like to take my time, but if I have to, I can do it quickly.

I had been living in San Diego and then moved to Scottsdale, Arizona. Then I got up the nerve to move to Los Angeles. I had been in L.A. for three months when I met Shay Mitchell. She found me through Instagram and has really helped my makeup career a lot.

The thing about Instagram is that it's become the only portfolio a makeup artist needs. I would say my clients, about 95 percent, reach out to me because they look at my work on social media. It's much easier for them to access me that way instead of emailing around these clunky portfolios.

From Shay, I met Gigi. She's such a rising sensation. I would definitely say I got really lucky, but it was also the social media that helped so much. The other part of being a makeup artist is that you have to be really comfortable with your clients. You're up in their faces and with them almost every single day. You're with them the majority of their work lives.

With Gigi, she honestly embodies that golden and bronze-y look, and she loves fresh skin. But she also loves glam sometimes. I try to encompass both. The fun part is she's a chameleon. I love going with a full look for wherever she's going. She likes makeup and she's OK with sitting awhile. A lot of stars or models might not be that way.

PATRICK'S SMOKY EYE TIPS

Starting point: I like doing eyes that look smoky when they are open but when you close your eyelid, it isn't too dark, so you still look fresh. I do that by emphasizing the drama in the lower lash line and outer crease, but I leave the center of the lid lighter. This brings light to the eyes and gives you a more wearable approach.

Colors: Maybe a couple years ago people weren't wearing color. But if you can get away with it, why not color? It's so much fun.

Product: I prefer cream eyeshadows; they look more expensive and rich. There are these Caviar Sticks by Laura Mercier that I love. The color payoff is more amazing. And it looks like it's a part of your eyelid instead of just sitting on the surface.

Here's How I Apply Them:
- Start with concealer as your lid base.
- Apply your powder eyeshadow next, keeping the center of the lid lighter.
- Apply your cream eyeshadow by putting it right on your lash line and then using a blending brush to blend the product out.
- For definition, use a darker color and then blend it upward into the brows.
- Add liner next. I prefer pencils because they blend into the lash line. Look for one that glides smoothly on the back of your thumb.
- Brush on mascara. Go for one that's not clumpy. I'm really loving the Gucci one because the brush really combs through every lash and the formula doesn't flake.
- If you're going for a full look, I like to add individual lashes. Ardell makes a great range. I use different lengths to create a more natural look and place them according to people's eye shape. If you want a more round eye look, place the longer lengths in the center of the eye. If you want a more cat or almond eye look, place them more at the outer corners.

LASHING OUT

Mascaras are as varied as the women featured in this book—that is, very.

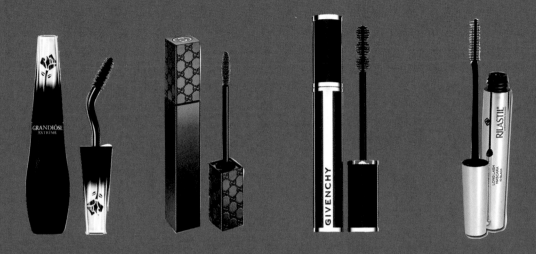

LANCÔME GRANDIÔSE EXTRÊME

With my nearly non-existent lash line, this angled wand works miracles for accenting my wimpy lashes. Those favoring a clean, minimal look might want to run the other way. The thick formula is all about the '60s mega-lash look. Viva Biba!

GUCCI INFINITE LENGTH

Model Lexi Boling and makeup artist Patrick Ta prefer the defining and separating capabilities of this wand.

GIVENCHY NOIR COUTURE 4 IN 1

Martha Stewart calls this wand, which looks like three stacked balls, "very cute." It also performs. "It makes your eyelashes look elongated," she says.

RILASTIL with VOLUMIZING EFFECT

"I have the best mascara in the business," Patricia Clarkson says of this Italian brand. "I hate to bring it out, because it's already so hard to find. It lengthens the lash and it stays, but it also comes right off."

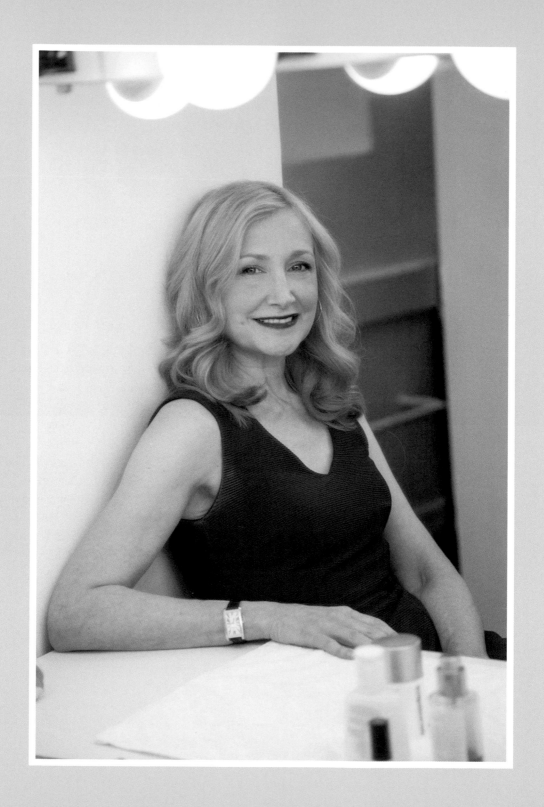

Patricia Clarkson

Actress

MAKEUP

I have four sisters. I was raised in a house of lipstick and hair curlers. They would laugh if they heard me giving you beauty tips. But if we happen to be home, we still like to do our hair and makeup together. I'm very specific about my makeup. I use Clé de Peau foundation. It's light but the coverage is beautiful. It doesn't dry me out. But you pay for it. I discovered it from another makeup artist. They're quite resourceful; they've seen so many types of faces and skin and they know a lot about the actress life and the special needs we might have. I also use an undereye stick by Shu Uemura that's amazing but hard to find. I was using Clé de Peau, but I switched to Chanel's translucent powder. For blush, there's a soft pink by Kevyn Aucoin that I really like.

I have all these expensive eye shadow palettes but I like Maybelline. I have a beautiful taupe and a gray. I use Sephora liquid liner in black and gray. They stopped making the gray, which kills me. I have the best mascara in the business. I hate to

bring it out, because it's already so hard to find. It's the volumizing mascara by Rilastil, this Italian brand. It lengthens the lash and it stays, but it also comes right off. Again, you have to pay for it.

And then lipstick, I have several. My favorite is Revlon Cherries in the Snow. My mother wears it; I wear it. I've worn it for a very, very long time—red lips have become my signature, and they're powerful. My mother taught me that. She was the president of the city council and ran New Orleans for years and years. She was a powerhouse of a woman. She wore red lipstick every day of her life.

I also own a beautiful Dior red. I just used a brand-new lipstick at Sephora that's incredible, a darker red by Bite Beauty. I only stay with reds in the blue undertone family. I have no tricks for helping it stay on. I just reapply. I have been known to turn a car around to get my lipstick.

If I'm going to be on stage or on the red carpet, I use Bobbi Brown Bronzing Powder in Golden Light. I probably need contour for my daily life, but I don't do it. I've always done my makeup for the stage. This play, *The Elephant Man*, is set in the 1880s, so the makeup isn't tremendous. I just keep a little more color—the Kevyn Aucoin or a MAC blush—in my face.

SKIN CARE

I try to use all-natural products as much as I can. I use Tom's soap. I also have Nature's Gate body wash. I generally like anything that has aloe vera in it. Kiehl's Creme de Corps is the best body lotion there is. It's incredible on the legs: It gives it such a sheen and it stays. It's really fabulous for every day, but also really great for red carpets for your arms and your legs.

Then, I wash my face with Cetaphil, and the toner I use is by Dr. Hauschka (it's just the classic facial toner, straight up). I've been using Cetaphil for a very long time: Don't fix what ain't broke. And of course, I use moisturizer. There's this amazing stuff called Power Rich by Dermalogica and it comes in little tiny tubes. That's my main moisturizer but I use Dermalogica products throughout. I used to use La Roche-Posay before, but a makeup artist told me I should try out Dermalogica and now I really love the line. Sometimes, I'll mix it up and use the Dermalogica Super Rich Repair. I'll also use the Multivitamin exfoliator, which is incredible. I'll use the Redness Relief, which has SPF 20, but not every day. I stay out of the sun. People are always like "Your skin, what's the secret?" Hats! Everybody knows I live in hats. I have a huge collection.

For night, I just use my Cetaphil and I also have a great makeup remover that's all-natural called No Tears! If I need it, there's a moisturizing mask by Dr. Hauschka that I really like. Then it's moisturizer and to bed.

FRAGRANCE

I have Stila Crème Bouquet. A man once told me I smelled like cookies. They used to sell it everywhere, but now I have to order it online.

HAIR

I use many shampoos and conditioners. It's good to change up products so your hair doesn't get used to something. I'll use everything from the beautiful olive conditioner and shampoo from Kiehl's—I love that—to Aveda to Redken's All Soft line. Or I'll just use John Frieda. I've had crazy thick hair since I was a child. It's gotten a little thinner now. It's naturally wavy and sometimes I get a blow out around the corner. Or I'll just put hot curlers in it. I'm a Southern girl. I've got lots of hot curlers.

This woman, Angie Elizalde, cuts my hair. She also does my hair for the red carpet. I have a few more layers in it right now. It looks better on me—it gave it swing.

I have several people who color my hair. I go around the corner to Jean Ferre, but then I also have a man, Manny Novoa, who has colored my hair for twenty-five years. My hair has been the same color forever: golden strawberry blonde. I've pretty much found what works for me. We play dress up so

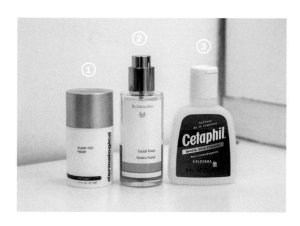

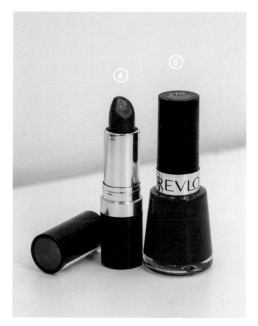

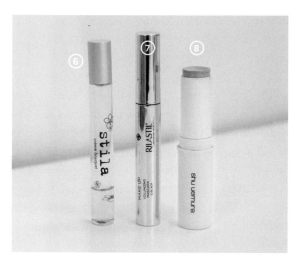

1 **Dermalogica**
Super Rich Repair

2 **Dr. Hauschka**
Facial Toner

3 **Cetaphil**
Gentle Skin Cleanser

4 **Revlon**
Cherries in the
Snow Lipstick

5 **Revlon**
Cherries in the Snow
Nail Enamel

6 **Stila** Crème Bouquet

7 **Rilastil**
Volumizing Mascara

8 **Shu Uemura**
Cream Cover Stick
Foundation

often, but sometimes, it's just easier to do what you know.

OTHER SERVICES

I'll occasionally get a facial. I know you do these interviews and people go to these fancy places. But I used to just go to this place on Greenwich Avenue called Janna Beauty. It's now closed. I'm not sure where my woman, Svetlana, moved to yet. For manicures and pedicures, I just go down the street. I get the essie classic red or Revlon Cherries in the Snow.

DIET AND FITNESS

I try to work out twice a week with a trainer. I walk a lot and I eat very good food. I'm gluten-free and dairy-free and I have been for many, many years.

When I have a show, I have to eat early. I have to eat a lot of protein and I'll probably do some protein shakes. For *The Elephant Man*, I have to wear a corset, so you know there's not much room in there. I won't be able to eat past four.

Rachel Roy

Fashion Designer

HAIR

Ted Gibson has been cutting my hair for years. If I bring in a tear or a picture of what I want, he'll just laugh at me. The reason he's laughing is because he knows me so well. He'll say: "C'mon Rachel, I know what you want." I have pretty heavy Indian hair, and he manages that well. He cuts in a way that makes your hair fuller and gives you layers but looks more effortless. I also like going to him because he's easy on the length. He doesn't chop too much off.

I've never had my hair dyed. I've never even had it highlighted. I'm not opposed to it. I'd actually like to try it. Having really dark hair, I do think highlights are nice, because it breaks it up.

My indulgence: scalp massages. I've been getting them for years with the same woman who comes to my house about once a week. I may not be the best person to ask on what to do with

wrinkles or what to do for your hair—I guess with my time, I just have my limits as to how much I can give to my face and hair—but I do believe in going to experts. It's part of the relaxation for me and it's like when you do yoga: It'll make you feel more centered and relaxed, so why not do it? I think women sometimes feel guilty for scheduling this stuff in, but it's important to take time out for yourself.

As far as styling, it's pretty simple. Recently, I found this powder that is texturizing and adds volume. It looks like a tiny baby powder—it's called Big Sexy Hair Powder Play—and it can travel with me everywhere. You put it in the roots of your hair and it really gives you that Gisele bedhead kind of beach-y look.

Otherwise, I don't even own a hair dryer. I don't know how to do hair. I do have a flat iron somewhere in the house, but my thirteen-year-old has stolen it from me. So I'm usually going

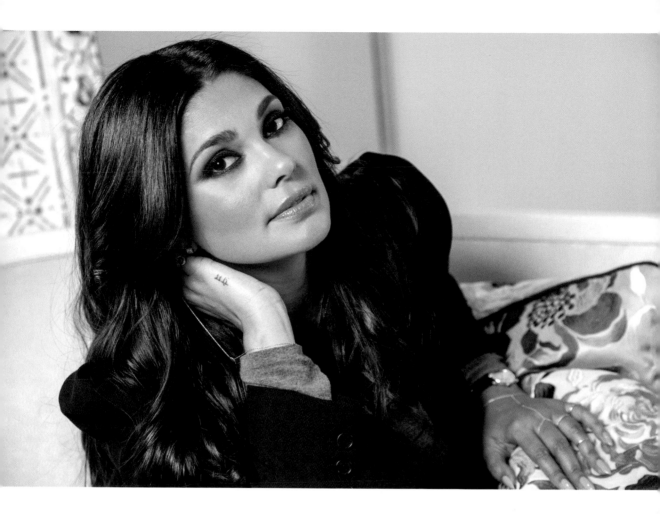

to do that messy hair look or a ponytail.

SKIN CARE

Recently, I started using this moisturizer called Dragon's Blood, which is by Rodial. Because my face is sensitive, I tend to be careful with what I use. But a makeup artist that I work with for events recommended I try this line and I've noticed a difference. It hydrates and plumps those lines, and all of that stuff that you want to prevent. There are lots of different products that go with it, like a mask and an eye gel that you put on for puffiness. I also use this Stemcell Super-Food Facial Oil from the same brand. It's good when you want extra moisture.

For cleanser, though, in the morning I'll just use Dove, the soap that I have in the shower. At night, I'll use a facial wipe from the drugstore for removing makeup. It's called Simple and it has no alcohol, no oil, no perfumes, and no dyes. Then I'll apply my Dragon's Blood routine.

MAKEUP

If it's just a day in the office, I won't use foundation or powder. I do love the Tom Ford Bronzing Powder. It's enough color for the cheeks to look youthful, fresh, and alive. It comes in a very thin elongated compact, so the mirror is bigger than most compacts, but it's still thin enough to travel with. I carry it with me everywhere.

I'm not great with lipstick during the day because it comes off so easily. I need a neutral color. Lately, I like Tom Ford's lipstick in Casablanca. There are some by Bobbi Brown that I also use, like Sandwash Pink and Tulle. It gives you color, but is not so difficult to manage.

I do lots of mascara. For me, that's something that wakes me up and makes me feel put together. I swear by Turbo-Lash. It has a battery in it and I put a few coats in the front and on the back of the lashes.

What I do love, though, are the small little tips I pick up, like the Indian smoky eye I do. It's great for covering wrinkles, and it's just so easy. The messier it is, the better. I use Bobbi Brown eyeliner because it's really soft and smudges great. I'll pair that with a Bobbi Brown smudge stick, which is kind of like an eyeshadow on a stick, in gray and blend that in. Usually I won't use jet-black shadow as it's too harsh. Gray works the best. Then, of course, I finish it off with the TurboLash.

FRAGRANCE

I love Red Roses by Jo Malone. It's a light and fresh scent. I'm a huge fan of the line's candles—I'm a big believer in all of the senses and getting to surround yourself with things that really make you happy— and I stumbled across this perfume. It's now my signature. I'll mix it with my Chanel No. 5 hand lotion, but that's usually more for the evenings.

OTHER SERVICES

I'm the type of person that if my toes and hands aren't done, I feel incomplete. That's the one thing that I can manage. I have someone come to my apartment in New York so that way I can still be by my kids. It takes about an hour and it's really relaxing. I usually have a red on my toes; I would say for the last twenty years almost. Chanel Rouge Rubis is kind of my go-to right now. For my hands, I've tried nail art before, but when I know I'm going to have a week where I have many things going on, I just go with a neutral. Then I don't have to think about what outfit. For the summer, the color would be in the nude family. This fall, I like this Chanel taupe-y gray called Frenzy. It goes with everything.

About once a month, I go to the Caudalie salon in the Plaza where I see Regine. It's about eighty minutes and it's half massage and half checking out the skin and seeing what's going on. She'll use this brush-light combo for anti-aging. I also try to go once a month to see Tracie Martyn. She has a lot of tools and lights to tighten and firm. I think these appointments are probably great preventatives. I'm turning forty soon, and for now, my beauty routine is to do the least possible, so it's good to have someone like Tracie, who zaps me back into place.

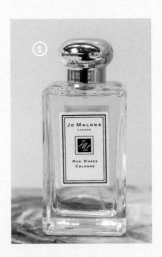

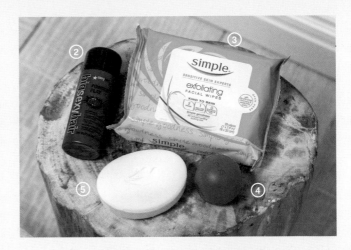

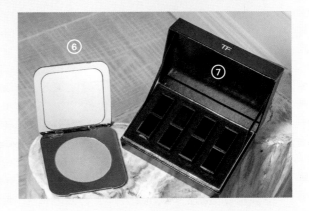

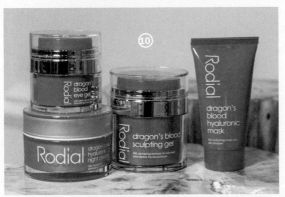

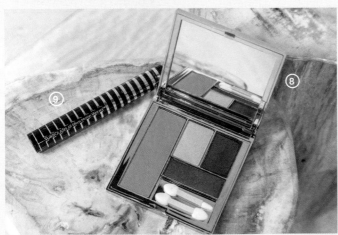

1 **Jo Malone**
Red Roses Cologne

2 **Big Sexy Hair**
Powder Play

3 **Simple** Exfoliating
Facial Wipes

4 **eos** lip balm

5 **Dove** Beauty Bar

6 **Tom Ford** bronzing
powder

7 **Tom Ford** lipstick set

8 **Aerin**
eyeshadow palette

9 **Estée Lauder**
TurboLash

10 **Rodial** Dragon's
Blood products

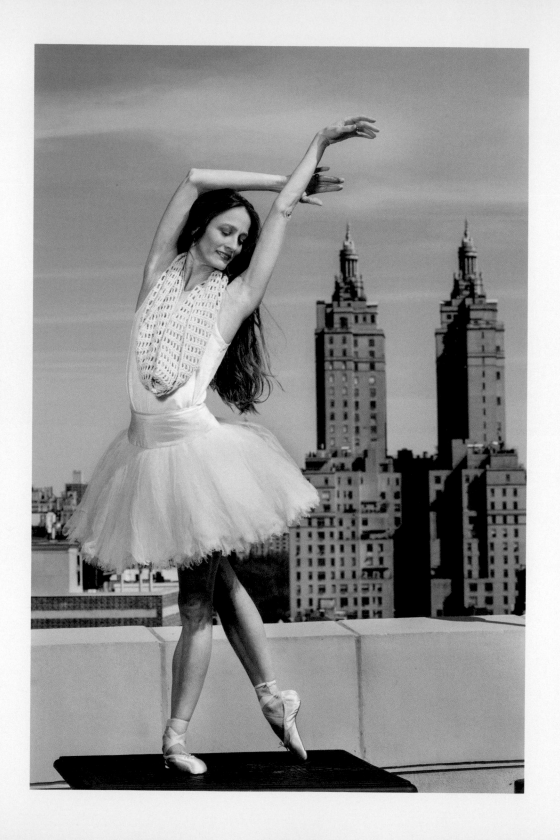

Julie Kent

Ballerina

DIET AND FITNESS

I've been dancing for so long, I don't really have any memories of not dancing. It's hard to think of it as exercise. The days off, I'm really resting. I get a chance to catch up on years of exhaustion and physical fatigue.

I did start doing Pilates after the birth of my son. I had a C-section, and I love how it's about keeping your core strong—your stomach supports your back which supports your hips which supports your knees and feet, which means you'll save yourself a lot of problems going forward.

And I've always had a really sound and healthy diet. My mom always made sure I had enough calories to sustain me when I was a teenager. Puberty is a vulnerable time for a dancer—really for any young woman. All of a sudden, you have a new body and you're in leotards and tights and looking at yourself in the mirror all day. There were young dancers who were only eating salads all the time. Well, they'd be starving by bedtime and eat a pint of ice cream. Those are just not good eating habits. My mother would make me a little steak and a potato and a salad. It's important to pass that on to my children and also what beauty means in the bigger picture. I received a note once from the famous Natalia Makarova. She said, essentially, beauty can save the world, what a big responsi-

84

bility you have on your shoulders. This concept has meant different things at different times in my life, but it's been constant in my purpose of ballet: the beauty of humanity that is so classically expressed in art and dance. But there is beauty in everything—if you look for it and find it in yourself, and if you contribute it to your world in any way you can. You don't have to be a ballet dancer.

SKIN CARE

Skin is important for a ballerina. During performance season, it's heavy makeup and sweating, repeatedly. It really takes a toll. So when I was seventeen, I had my first facial with Simone France in NYC. One of the dancers in the company told me about her, and I went to her for years. She is about eighty-five years old and retired now. I still use her products though. She has this regimen that involves using a moisturizer and scrub and then a cleanser. You moisturize again after. There are a couple of other products I really like, especially if I have breakouts, which I still do. Mario Badescu has a Drying Lotion that you can dab on when you have a pimple, and I like Dr. Hauschka's Day Oil that normalizes skin. Simone has a rich lotion, which I use for taking off makeup. If I feel like I need something foaming, then I'll use Mario Badescu, and he's got so many different ones, like the Glycolic Foaming Cleanser.

In the shower, right now I'm using this wonderful body wash by Antica Farmacista. It's rose and peony—a really lovely floral. My daughter and I really go through it. She's only five, but she likes to smell good too.

MAKEUP

I have three stages of makeup wearing. There's my daily, which is just going to the studio and working. It's very light makeup and I use the Make Up For Ever concealer and tinted moisturizer with SPF by NARS. Because I have really sensitive skin around my eyes, I only use Aveda mascara. Sometimes when I use other brands, my eyelids get puffy and swollen. As far as lipstick, well, NARS has got a really great Velvet Gloss Lip Pencil. It's fast and not too makeup-y and gives you color. I always like to have something I can share with my daughter, too, so I might have some really sheer and pale Bite Beauty lip glosses around. Bite Beauty is edible, so I feel like it's relatively safe.

Then, there's my midrange makeup, if I'm attending an event or doing a presentation or going to a meeting. If I need more, then I use this wonderful palette by Eve Pearl. There are three eye shadows and two blush colors there, and it's small enough that I can take it with me. I also really like the Bobbi Brown Shimmer Brick. My mom bought it for me a long time ago, and it's something I use occasionally when I need just a little bit of color.

For the stage, it's a heavy cake foundation. You have to put it on with a sponge—we're talking complete coverage. Then comes powder and cake eyeliner with a brush and

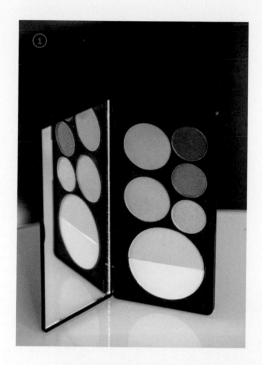

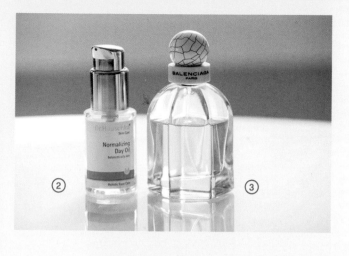

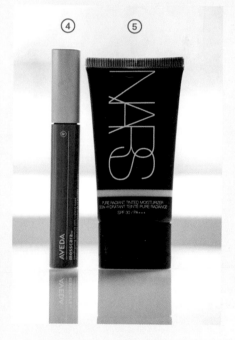

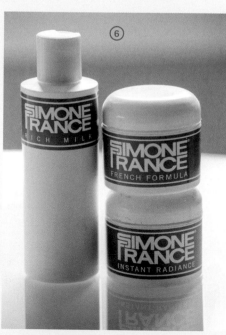

1 **Eve Pearl**
palette

2 **Dr. Hauschka**
Normalizing Day Oil

3 **Balenciaga**
perfume

4 **Aveda** mascara

5 **Nars**
Pure Radiant
Tinted Moisturizer

6 **Simone France**
Rich Milk, French
Formula, and Instant
Radiance

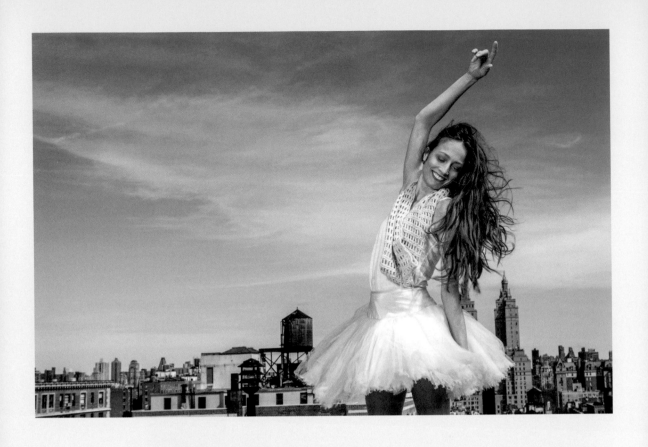

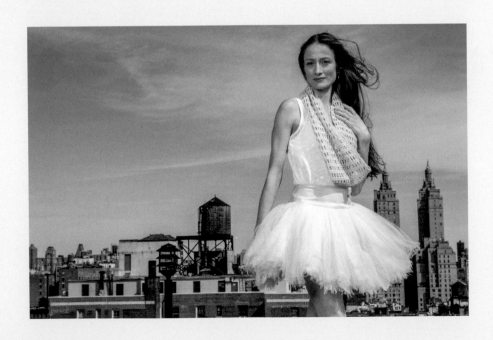

water—you have to do very big lines around the eyes and maybe some contouring. And we always wear eyelashes. Eyes need to be expressive on the stage.

FRAGRANCE

I love the classic Balenciaga fragrance. I discovered it at the duty-free shop about five years ago when I danced in Moscow. Just a couple years before that, my ballet mistress, who was like my second mother, passed away. She was British and had this fabulous British accent and I just remember her saying "Balenciaga" during a conversation. I don't even remember what she was talking about, but I just remember hearing it so clearly that when I saw it at duty-free, it reminded me of her. Of course, I love what's in the bottle too.

HAIR

I actually was a Pantene girl and did Pantene commercials about ten to fifteen years ago. The classic shampoo is really good. And this is my natural color—thank god. Although, I'm looking closely at my older sister to see when I'll start needing to cover grays. She's five years older than me and so far, so good.

For styling products, I love Sally Hershberger's 24K Root Envy. I have very long hair and it's fine, and so it does tend to hang a bit if it's not plumped up a little bit at the roots. I don't get my hair cut that often. Long hair is certainly not mandatory when you're a ballerina, but it's very useful as a principal dancer because you have to wear your hair down for certain acts and just to make different beautiful shapes like buns and twists for certain characters. Otherwise, you have to use pieces and it gets complicated.

SERVICES

For me, pedicures are a huge part of maintaining your feet as a dancer. Our feet are our tools. I highly recommend a pumice stone to get the calluses. You need the calluses to a certain point, but don't let them build up too much. And it's also a source of vanity for me! I don't want to be caught in the summer wearing sandals and look down and see these unpleasant toes. I just go to the neighborhood salons or I do it a lot myself. I like the polishes from Whole Foods like Mineral Fusion. I like darker colors on my toes, but when you're performing, you can't wear any colors on your fingers.

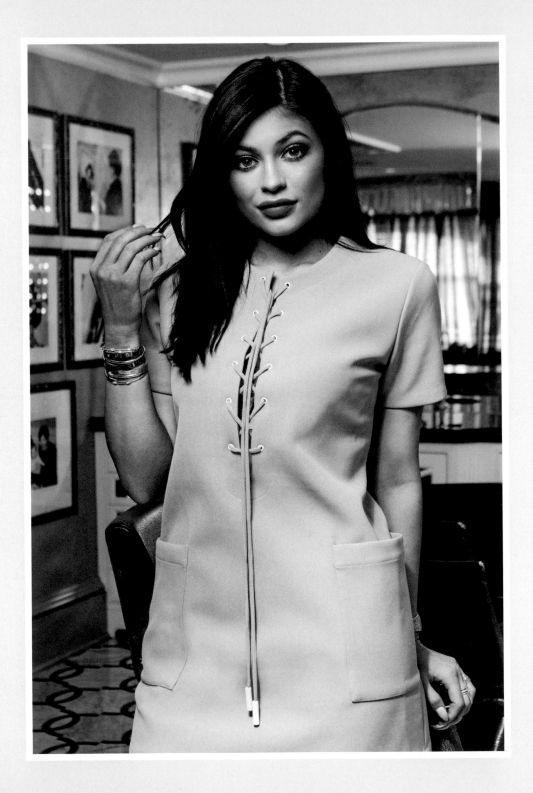

Kylie Jenner

Founder of Kylie Cosmetics

MAKEUP

If I'm going to see people, I won't wear heavy makeup. It's not attractive on me. When you see those pictures on my Instagram, they are usually for when I am doing a photo shoot or an interview. Every time I get my makeup professionally done, I take a photo.

I do love lashes and lip liner and a light foundation and bronzer though. My usual go-to is the Charlotte Tilbury Light Wonder foundation. You can still see my skin through it. I'm not down with heavy foundation all the time. Then, I use NARS Orgasm blush. For my lashes, I like to go to CVS and explore all the falsies. I used to be obsessed with heavy lashes, but now I just want to find something super clean and light. I like the Wispies ones. Mascara, I've been using Lancôme Hypnôse Drama. And Anastasia Beverly Hills has this contour kit that's just easy and everything is there. The woman who founded it, Anastasia Soare, also does my eyebrows—she does all my sisters' brows. For bronzer, I've been using the Kardashian bronzer. I use it in the hollow of my cheekbones, the sides of my head, my nose, and under my chin. I really love the Anastasia concealer; I like my concealer to have a bit of pink in it because it brightens the area up. For powder, I use the Bobbi Brown yellow powder that they have. I like yellow because it cancels out any red and also it works really well with my spray tan color.

If I'm doing a lip, it depends on what I'm feeling for the day. I like lip liners over lipsticks. I have so many of them from so many different brands, so I just pick the color that works. I'm in the middle of creating my own lip kit, and I'm doing my three favorite colors: nude, a sepia color, and a true brown. I'm super quick at this now. I could do this in ten minutes. But if I'm doing lashes, it'll take a few extra minutes.

If I do amp it up, I usually go for a lot of illuminator. I love to be super shiny, like that strobing trend that's happening on Instagram. Anastasia has an awesome highlighter —I love the gold one. It's not too crazy and not too subtle, where you have to do too much to make it show.

SKIN CARE

We have a family dermatologist: Christie Kidd in Beverly Hills. My sister Kendall had really bad acne when she was younger and she really cleared it up. I thought, "Well if she cured Kendall, I should start to visit her." It's been years now. I use her face wash in the morning and my sister Khloe taught me to wear sunscreen. I use one by TiZO$_3$. It doesn't really smell like sunscreen, which I like, and it's tinted. If I wake up in the morning and have to run somewhere, I'll just put that on solo. I use this all-natural moisturizer called Mimosa Blossom Dream Cream. I like

to find new pure things. I have sensitive skin and it's super dry so a lot of stuff irritates me. There's this grocery store by me called Erewhon that has all these vitamins and natural shampoos and conditioners and stuff—that's where I found it. I like to go look around there for natural oils or new products. For eye cream, I love the Kiehl's avocado eye cream.

At night, I'll use the Neutrogena makeup remover wipes. I do the same moisturizer, and I also found these masks at Sephora that all my friends are using. I'm obsessed with them.

HAIR

I used to wash my hair every day and then a lot of people told me that wasn't good for your hair so now I try for every other day. I like the Moroccanoil shampoo and conditioner. I used to have really thick hair with a lot of body, but not anymore. About a year and a half ago, I cut it off and then I kept bleaching it and dying it blue so that damaged it a bit. Then on my seventeenth

birthday, I shaved half my head so my underneath is still growing back. I'm waiting for it to grow out, but it's still only 50 percent there.

My natural hair color is like a brown with a reddish tint. Right now, it's jet black. I can't have brown hair for some reason—I don't think it goes with my skin tone. The second I see it turn brown in the sun, I dye it black—the blacker the better. I get my hair cut by Priscilla Valles. She also puts my extensions in. Daniel Moon dyes Nicole Richie's hair and I love the color she had—this silvery purple. He did my blue color. Next, though, I want to see Tracey Cunningham because I want to go blonde soon. She's supposed to be the best with blondes.

I usually style my own hair unless I have an event. I always wear my hair down. I'm not comfortable yet with wearing my hair up, although I do want to experiment.

OTHER SERVICES

I love my spray tans. I go to Jimmy Coco. If I just want to be

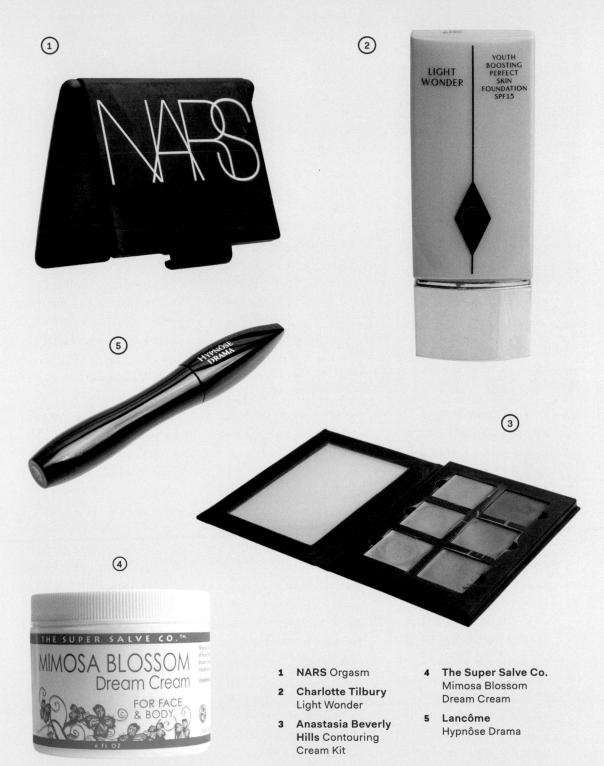

1 **NARS** Orgasm

2 **Charlotte Tilbury** Light Wonder

3 **Anastasia Beverly Hills** Contouring Cream Kit

4 **The Super Salve Co.** Mimosa Blossom Dream Cream

5 **Lancôme** Hypnôse Drama

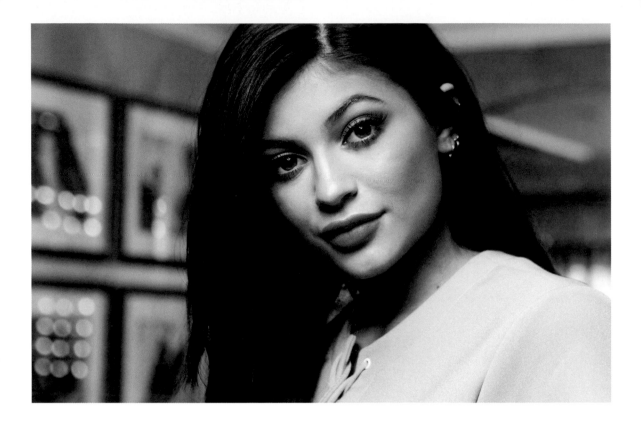

tan for one night, sometimes I use the Sally Hansen leg spray. Kimmie Kyees does my nails. I do love my acrylics and long nails, but right now I'm into simple light colors for summer.

I still do Juvéderm for my lips. I go to Dr. Ourian in Beverly Hills. He's the best and he's super natural about it. I was going to somebody before and it was just looking crazy. Also, I would recommend anyone who gets it done to go for the one that lasts only about two to four months. It's annoying to keep going back but then you have the option

of stopping it. Also, Juvéderm tends to make your lips dry. I try to do a lot of sugar lip scrubs and any lip moisturizer. I like Aquaphor.

FRAGRANCE

I don't really wear perfume. I use Victoria's Secret sometimes, they have this Coconut Passion spray, but fragrances can give me a bit of a headache.

DIET AND FITNESS

My sister Kourtney had her third baby recently and she is

on a workout health kick to get her body back. She lives up the street, so I'll join her for a trainer session sometimes. I also started going to this nutritionist, because I was having a bad reaction to dairy. I feel like it made me gain a lot of weight. I've now cut out dairy and it's helping me get back in shape, which is just working out and watching what I eat. Every time I get hungry for a snack during the day, I like to have the Justin's Almond Butter packets. It's easy.

MARIO DEDIVANOVIC
SOCIAL MEDIA'S INFLUENCE on BEAUTY

It's undeniable Instagram, YouTube, and, more recently, Snapchat have changed the world of makeup. Not only has social media created an insatiable thirst for color products, but it's also become more inclusive of a wide variety of beauty looks. Though there are a dizzying array of influencers today, I still think of Kim Kardashian and her makeup artist Mario Dedivanovic as the early originators of a certain Instagram aesthetic: exaggerated, defined, and not shy of a full-face application. Interestingly, when this look took hold, there was a counterpoint in the editorial beauty circles I traveled in.

Full glamour was being celebrated on the one hand and yet many of my peers were choosing to go with the "no makeup, makeup" look. Suffice it to say, Instagram beauty, which came to be associated with heavy use of foundation, false lashes, heavy brows, and wild colors, became controversial. When I spoke with Mario, I was surprised where he came out on the debate. Then again, unlike a Patrick Ta, whose career was formed and bred on social media, Mario's career started on a much more traditional foundation.

Where he's coming from...

I've done everything in the past fifteen years. I worked in retail and then I was assisting makeup artists and then I began working for brands. When I was assisting on fashion shoots, I was always very conscious about what I was doing. To be successful in fashion, it's difficult. There are only a very few at the top. So I made the decision to pursue celebrity. I started seeking out photographers who were shooting more celebrity-type stuff and then working with more socialites. It started with smaller celebrities like Miss Universe and then word would get around.

Discovering social media...

When I started my career, there was no Instagram or Twitter. I remember getting on Twitter when it started but then not doing anything with it. When Instagram came along, I didn't even know how to use it for a long time. I was actually late to Instagram compared to what everybody else did. I wasn't thinking at the time that it would change the beauty industry, which it has significantly.

But then I started teaching master makeup classes. I thought Instagram might be an amazing way to promote my master classes. It was becoming such a big thing, and I saw the industry start to change. Makeup artist rates were going down. The influence was shifting. But how do I find a way to stay on top of what I was doing and to gain a following like what these bloggers and YouTubers had?

I made a conscious effort to learn about the platform. It was a lot of time devoted daily to figuring out what to post and what kinds of posts would draw the most followers.

Learning how to attract followers...

I never posted anything so crazy. I still have to remain someone that other aspiring artists look up to. Because of that, I don't go overboard. I teach the techniques, and then everyone kind of takes that method and goes overboard. I'm more in-between.

A lot of stuff I post is not necessarily the most beautiful or tasteful, but you have to give or take a little bit. I know my followers like a certain type of makeup but I also put out what I like. It's a fine line.

You also have to keep up a constant stream of content. I will do at least one to two posts a day and sometimes even twelve.

On working with Kim Kardashian...

I got hired to do her makeup on a magazine cover about ten years ago. We've really grown together. She has become a major influence around the world. I know that better maybe than anyone else. I hear about it and see it every day. It's really fascinating, even to me. To this day, she's still the number one requested beauty look around the world. And can you imagine the number of YouTube re-creations of her that are out there?

No matter what people think of her on a personal level, there's no denying she influences beauty.

It's hard for me even to pinpoint why. I could spend days talking about that and there's not an exact answer. There's some relatability to her. She has a reality show and she puts her whole life out there. Normal celebrities, you see them on the stage or in a movie and that's it. With Kim, you see her shopping or doing everyday things. That must have something to do with it, although I'm not sure.

Then there's the fact she is absolutely gorgeous. She's a glam girl. She brought this entire glam look into the global beauty space and then she showed everyone how she did it. Before, no celebrities and no makeup artists were really putting the tricks of the trade out there. So women would see this beautiful makeup and it was very unachievable.

Kim and I, we would start posting pictures of our routine, such as contouring, etc. At the same time, I started teaching these tricks in my master classes. All these YouTubers and influencers would come to the classes and they would do the look for their own channels and blow it up. It's fascinating how something might become a global trend.

They started calling me the "King of Contour," and I hated it for so long. Then I started getting really big-paying jobs because of it. Well, if that's what I am, so be it.

The thing is, I've always done the same amount of contour. Contour will always be around. We'll always want to shape and define the face. But the extreme hype will slowly go away. And I'm honestly pushing a cleaner look right now.

But that's not the case with what I'm seeing on the street often. Drag queen makeup is not anything new. The social media people are doing it in a very drastic way because they get more likes.

How social media has influenced beauty...

Some people would say social media is the worst thing that's ever happened to beauty. Now when you go to an agency that represents makeup artists, one of the first questions they ask you is how many followers do you have. It's because we make money from brands and brands want followers. It's not just your day rate anymore. The influencers are a perfect example. They've started to cut into what the traditional makeup artists do. Thankfully, I have a found a way I can do both.

Where social media is going today...

I don't know where it's all going. I think about it sometimes. I don't think it'll be possible to keep going at the rate it's going now. I am paying attention to what's going on. Snapchat is really, really big, especially with the younger audience. Also, I've noticed sometimes I'll sell more of a product when I put it on Snapchat.

Social media is now a full-time job. Between Snapchat and Instagram and Facebook as well, there's so much to do in a day. But it's tough to tell what's going to be next. When Periscope first came out, they said it was the next big thing, I jumped on, and then it kind of died.

Whatever it is, I don't think Instagram's influence is going to last years and years. Perhaps the power will gear back toward celebrity makeup artists.

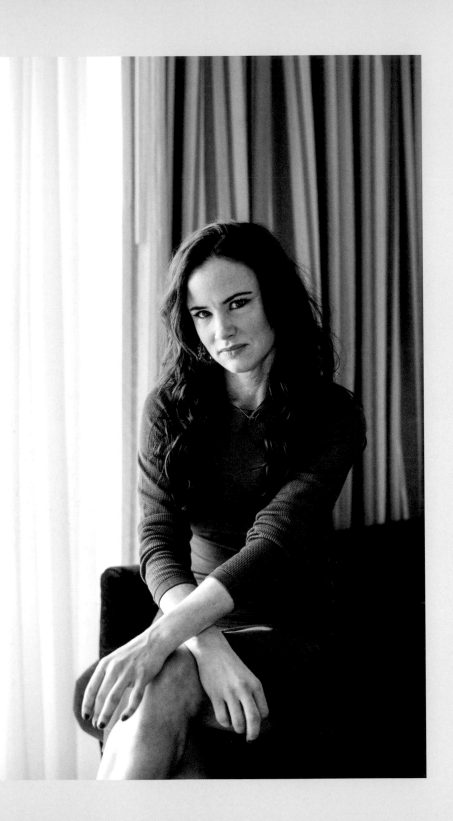

Juliette Lewis

Actress

MAKEUP

My eyebrows are a mess. I must explain. I was born with very strange eyebrows that are from my dad. They're skinny; they're dodgy. I don't know that I can be somebody to rep how to do great eyebrows. But I fill them in with a chocolate brown NARS pencil.

I actually did a photo shoot with François Nars like twenty years ago when he was first starting his makeup line and I really liked the products. I still use the NARS lip gloss. I like something that matches my own lip color, so roses are good. I get whatever lip balm at Whole Foods. Right now, it's Burt's Bees, and I like anything with vitamin E. Nowadays, I don't want a tan, but I do love blushes in colors that give you that whole sun-kissed thing. I don't wear any foundation unless I have to do a photo shoot or something. Then they always put the Giorgio

Armani Luminous Silk one on me; whoever discovered that formula must be really celebrating.

For nighttime, I tend to do my eyes. Wearing red lipstick sure is exciting, but man is it hard to get it to stay on. So I've always been about my eyes. To make them smoky, I use a brush. NARS has a great palette, and I also like one by Sigma, which has all these iridescent colors—it's called Spellbinding. I don't use mascara. Here I am telling you I'm as real as you can get with all that natural stuff, but then I am into fake lashes. There's a revelation! I have to give a shout out to my lash girl, Sandi Schroeder. She's the best. Just to be clear, I don't do *those* types of lashes—the ones that are so fake that are on this woman whose name we all know. They look really real. Sandi is fantastic; she uses surgical glue for each lash, which is great because I have really sensitive eyes, and they last for about two weeks. And we get to chat about boys while she's doing it—it's so fun. It's especially great for when I'm shooting *Secrets and Lies*, because I'm completely androgynous and get to wear almost no makeup at all, so a little bit of eyelashes is nice.

SKIN CARE

As I get older, everything is less. I wash my face, often with just water. Sometimes, I'll use a natural line called Nyou by Raw Beauty that my makeup artist Dana Michelle Hamel makes. Other than that, my skin regimen is so boring. I'm really into coconut oil for everything. I cook it, eat it, put it in my hair, and use it as body lotion. I put it on my face too—day cream, night cream, whatever. I love the smell—it reminds me of the beach. I'm not particular on what brand as long as it's organic. I discovered it because it's good for cooking and I grew up with a mother who was super into health food. Sometimes, I'll use this other really lightweight skin moisturizer called Klarif. My skin likes it, and I have really sensitive skin. I only wear SPF if I'm going to the beach—then it's one by Alba Botanica.

FRAGRANCE

I'm not a store-bought-scent person. I like fragrances that smell edible. I love coconut and vanilla and mango. I get this natural scented oil at Whole Foods called coco mango. Or I love lavender. Like I have the lavender body lotion by Alba Botanica.

HAIR

When I was on the road for my band, I had blue hair—loved it. This was years ago, before Katy Perry and everyone went blue and it went mainstream. I like to say I kicked it off. I would actually do it myself whenever I landed in a city. I've used Manic Panic and fans would bring me hair color! I would blend blue and aqua to make turquoise. I've left a few hotel sinks blue— like a Smurf exploded.

Right now, though, my hair is a rich brown, which is pretty much my natural hair color. It's boring. It's funny because now I'm contracted to a TV show, I can't really touch my hair. I've been dreaming of a little Louise Brooks bob that I had a hundred years ago, but I have to wait to see if this show gets picked up. To wash, I use Jāsön shampoo. It makes my hair full and voluminous. I also use Kenra Dry Texture Spray and again with the coconut oil, I put it on the ends of my hair.

SERVICES

I am always on the quest for the greatest masseuse. But I more often get bad massages than good ones, so I've started to avoid it. The best massages are from my man—he services me! But I'm not saying my man's name. People will find out soon enough.

DIET AND FITNESS

Everybody here is obsessed with fat. I'm not. I've always been a little person. (To say skinny is weird; it has so many connotations.) I'm pretty healthy diet-wise, but I'm not fanatical. I eat more for sustenance and comfort and pleasure, although I *love* butter. Otherwise, I'm pretty boring—a lot of protein and vegetables. I also take supple-

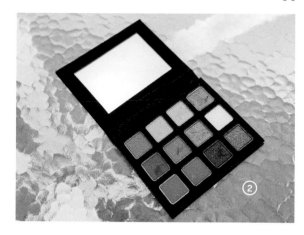

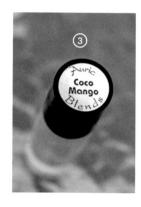

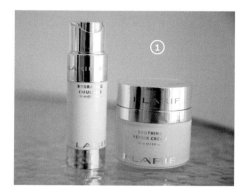

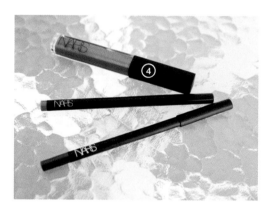

1 **Klarif**
Hydrating Emulsion,
Soothing Repair
Cream

2 **Sigma** Brilliant &
Spellbinding Palette

3 **Auric Blends**
Coco Mango

4 **NARS**
lip gloss, eyebrow
pencil, eyeliner

ments: these powder vitamins from my chiropractor, Dr. Stephen Price—you drink them. I love a place here called Glow Bio and I live on the almond milk coffee and juices at Pressed Juicery, which is right near my house.

When I was younger I took dance and gymnastics. Somewhere, that lives in my muscle memory. Also, I've always been physical in my acting and music. But after years of touring and doing five shows a week, I stopped about four years ago, and I got depressed and didn't know why. That's when I took up running. I realized I had to sweat and exert energy for my mental health. I also go to a class that I will scream and shout about because I love it so much. It's Barry's Bootcamp and I drag myself there every morning in whatever state I'm in and just listen and follow the trainer. Don't let the name scare you. I always leave there feeling elated.

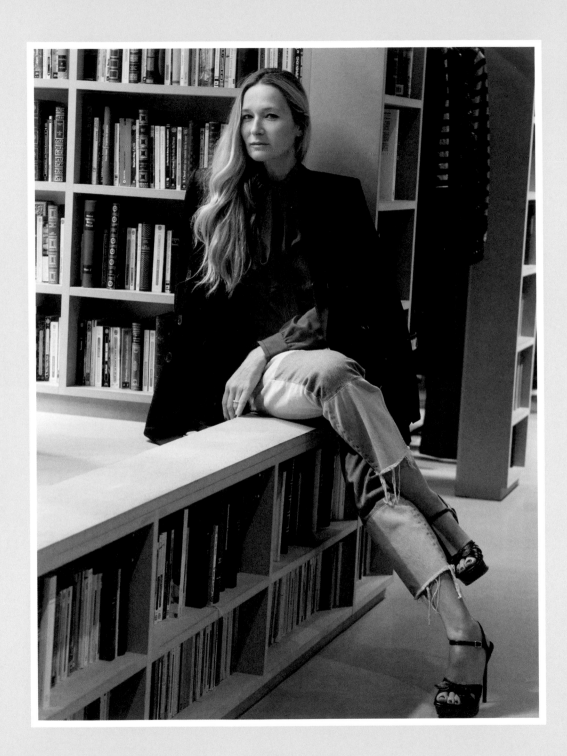

Julie de Libran

Fashion Designer, Sonia Rykiel

SKIN CARE

I wash my face at night. I've been told you shouldn't use soap in the morning—it's too aggressive. Obviously, when I take my shower, I put my head in the water, but I don't use soap. After the shower, I use a tonic by my epidermist, Joelle Ciocco. Her products are really good and quite natural and the smell is fantastic. You get hooked. I've been going at least since I moved back to Paris—so since 2008.

Then I use a complex serum with vitamin A that you put on before you put on your cream. It's fantastic. It's a little bit shiny but it absorbs and nourishes your skin in depth. I've been told I have very thin skin and quite delicate too. I need to keep my skin moisturized. I put a cream on top of that.

At night, I'll use one of her cleansers, which are really, really light. Again, they're not aggressive. I've tried many, many things—when I go to New York I've tried peels, and when I was in Korea I tried all the beauty products there, which are quite forward-thinking—but this is what suits me. My skin is not uniform and actually I get spots or redness in some places so having something not so strong works. One thing I've learned more recently is taking different vitamins to help nourish the skin. You can go to the French pharmacies here and find a beauty supplement. I find if I take it regularly, my skin is moisturized from the inside and it looks as if I've gone on holiday.

OTHER SERVICES

Joelle Ciocco has great girls who work for her and she has some who will go to your home. That's quite good for my schedule. I have to say it's such a luxury to have your trainer or this type of beauty service at home. So if I can do it, I try to organize as much as I can to happen at home.

I also have a great girl who does nails that comes to the house. She came this weekend; right now I have a really short nail in a deep red. It's so much maintenance to be a woman. It can be really hard. I asked my husband the other day if he liked my hair this way or that way. He's like, "Oh I just like it natural." Ha! You think this is natural?

MAKEUP

I don't wear a lot but I do put on a BB cream as a base. I like the one from REN because it's very light. And then I usually do just my eyes. I discovered this liquid liner that's so easy to use. It's from Charlotte Tilbury. And then on top, because

I like a black eye with a kind of smudged look, I'll use a Chanel or Sisley liner. I have different tricks depending on my day or mood. The Sisley one is good for a party or dinner. It's very thick and it also comes in a midnight blue that's pretty.

We just did a collaboration with Lancôme; I mostly use the eye palette—there's one that has that midnight blue that I love. My eye color is blue but it turns green or gray depending on what I wear. I'll do a blush or a lip if I'm going out because I'm making more of an effort. But if it's every day, I've been using the RMS Living Luminizer for years with nothing on the cheeks. I use it under and on the sides of my eyes.

FRAGRANCE

For me, it's very important. The gesture of putting on perfume, I love it. One of my closest friends is a nose and she's made a personal perfume for me, which is wonderful. But I also use one she made for Prada, which is actually the men's cologne. I like it because

it's not as sugary or as sweet as some of the perfumes out there. It smells like soap.

HAIR

I've been using David Mallett products—they're fantastic. He's also been cutting my hair lately. My hair is so long and he's so meticulous that I don't have to get it cut so much now because it grows out so well. I also get the head massages at his salon, which are amazing. It's really good if your hair is dry. I go to someone else for my color. I've been going to him for years; I'm quite what you call *fidèle*. His name is Jean. He used to be one of the Christophe Robin colorists but now he's independent. I just follow him around.

DIET AND FITNESS

I have to pay attention to diet and fitness. Diet, I always try to be attentive. I can be strict sometimes but sometimes I can also really just indulge. I'm vegetarian. I try to not have sugar—that's the worst thing for me. And then I exercise. If

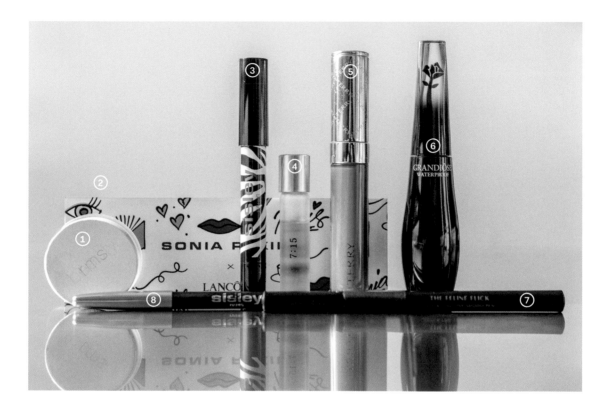

I'm exercising, then sometimes I can have cheese and bread and wine at dinner. I also exercise for my head; it's a way to liberate and get positive energy. I try to run once a week. I do Pilates on the reformer machine. I do Ashtanga or vinyasa yoga. And I have a new trainer I discovered just before the summer who is making me do things I hate, which I did at my American high school, like squats and things like that. In France, and all of Europe really, things are changing. There are so many trainers and gyms now.

1 **RMS** Living Luminizer

2 **Sonia Rykiel x Lancôme** eye palette

3 **Sisley Paris** eyeliner

4 **Uka** 7:15 nail oil

5 **By Terry** lip gloss

6 **Lancôme** Grandiose Waterproof Mascara

7 **Charlotte Tilbury** The Feline Flick

8 **Sisley Paris** eyeliner

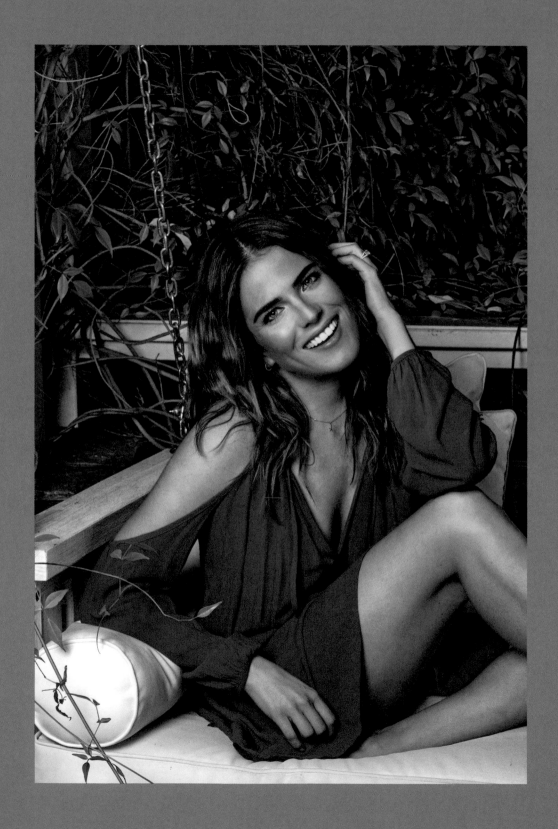

Karla Souza

Actress

DIET AND FITNESS

Do you ever meet anyone who doesn't pay attention to diet and fitness? I live in a world where a focus on diet and fitness is the new normal. Right now, I'm training for a triathlon but I also go to Hot 8 Yoga—there's one in Santa Monica—for the Yin yoga and the Bikram-like class. Anytime I have a photo shoot, I feel like going to hot yoga can help flush things out.

And I don't know anyone in my life that doesn't have a diet—and by that, I mean a regime of eating. Nowadays, we're so aware and conscious of everything. Whoever in this industry says they're not paying attention to diet, they're lying. My nutritionist is John Brandy. He helped me for *Jacob's Ladder*—I was playing a character that required me to lose weight and almost be unhealthy looking. It's also helpful to have somebody get me back on track the right way. You have to be careful you don't get a bad relationship with food. Now with the triathlon, he also helps me out and adds to my knowledge of food.

I also think there needs to be more said about what it takes to look a certain way. I did this *GQ* shoot and when I posted it to Instagram, people were saying "#bodygoals." I was like, "No, no, no. This is unsustainable." There were the two months of completely starving your body and it's not right for women to think that this is what "normal" is. It's important to say what took place behind it.

Of course, I have pressure to look a certain way, but that's not normal. For a sex scene, it would blow your mind what people would do for just that one day of shooting. But people watch and may think that's what normal looks like, when it's really not. It's a tricky thing. We're on network TV and people expect something when they think celebrity or actor/actress. If you don't diet and work out like crazy to look a certain way, you also get all these hate messages about being fat. But I'd like to point out how it's all relative. Our society values self-control and discipline because we live in a place of abundance. But places that are poorer, they value curves more. It's a social thing that's hard to change.

SKIN CARE

It depends if I have a break-out. If I feel like I'm having a breakout, there's a tea tree oil face wash—it's actually Trader Joe's— that's helped me when I have really oily skin. Other-wise, I'll use the Hydra Total 5 gel face wash from L'Oréal. I'm an ambassador for them. It does just enough to feel clean without being drying. I also use the toner from the same line and the moisturizer too. I like using the same line if I'm

going to layer products. I have faith in the fact—misplaced or not!—that since it's from the same line, the chemicals in the products should be used that same way.

I do change it up some-times when I feel like my skin needs a reboot. First Aid Beauty has a red clay mask and a mattifying gel that mini-mizes the appearance of pores, which I use occasionally. When I'm really dry—I've been based in L.A. now for the last two years and it's very dry out here—there's Kate Somerville Goat Milk cleanser that's super gentle. I also love using the Kate Somerville ExfoliKate and her acne treat-ment EradiKate, which can be really funny looking when you're putting it on because it goes on pink. I also use the DermalQuench retinol from her line for nighttime and matching eye cream.

I have freckles and I don't look great when I'm suntanned. I have a sunscreen from Kate Somerville that helps. But now with the triathlon training, I'm swimming in the ocean all the time, so there goes that.

MAKEUP

When I was younger, I was teased a little bit about my eyebrows, so it's funny now that it's become an "in" thing. I remember growing up, my dad would point to Charlotte Casiraghi and say, "See, she has big brows. You don't want to pluck them." I would pro-test, but I never did pluck.

Now I have them threaded at Brow Mantra, which is near me in Santa Monica. I do it about once a month. When I'm on the show, the makeup artist will use an ash-colored brow powder. I was also recently on a shoot for the *InStyle México* ten-year anni-versary cover and the makeup artist used this dark brown pencil. I thought it was way too strong in real life, but in the picture, I thought it looked amazing and framed my face in a really cool way.

Because I wear makeup all day for work, whenever I don't work, not wearing any is a luxury. I'm all for women us-ing makeup, but I'm also all for women not wearing makeup. I do carry that Benefit liquid

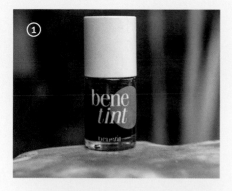

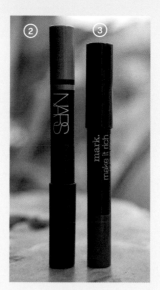

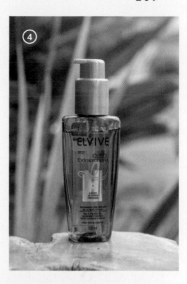

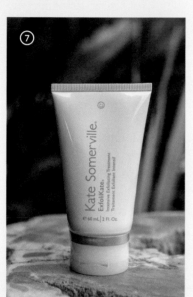

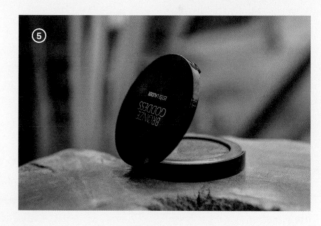

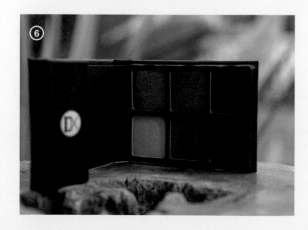

1 **Benefit** Benetint

2 **NARS** lip pencil

3 **Mark**
   Make It Rich
   lip pencil

4 **L'Oréal**
   Elvive

5 **Estée Lauder**
   Bronze Goddess

6 **Viseart**
   Theory Palette II

7 **Kate Somerville**
   ExfoliKate

stain. I use the stain everywhere. Because of my skin tone and eye color—they're blue—it makes everything pop. I'll do a little L'Oréal Butterfly mascara and with my brows, it's fine for day.

Whenever I go out or am in a wedding, there's this Airflash foundation by Dior that's really cool. It's a little cold when it comes out and it feels like there's a little mini de-puffing action happening. Who knows, it may be in my head. Or sometimes, I just love the L'Oréal Colour Riche 135, which is a great red. When I was younger, I would feel like I would have to do my whole face. But I've learned I can't use too much makeup with my features; I have to pick one thing. Otherwise it swallows my whole face up.

HAIR

I use the Total Repair 5 line of shampoo and conditioner by L'Oréal—I work with the brand on haircare. I also use a cream-based oil from L'Oréal Elvive. It's the same conditioner that I use when my hair is damp and I leave it in so it won't dry out. It'll help the hair stay hydrated and not crispy. When I wake up in the morning or need extra shine, I'll put the Elvive oil on my mid to lower ends.

My hair color: I just did a fiery red for *Jacob's Ladder*. Tracey Cunningham at Mèche, she did my coloring. I go to Adir Abergel, who also did my hair for the *InStyle* cover, for haircuts. With them, I'm good. After a color, I try to not shampoo as much. I usually only wash about once or twice a week. Now, my hair is back to a brown, but for *How to Get Away with Murder*, they really liked the red color, so they wanted to add a little bit of that in the show. So now it's brown but with traces of red at the ends.

FRAGRANCE

My husband is allergic to perfume. When he's away, I really like the DKNY Women one. When he's around, I've noticed I can wear the Satsuma Body Mist from The Body Shop. He just thinks I smell like an orange. I have to use really natural-smelling things—nothing fancy.

OTHER SERVICES

I went recently to Burke Williams. There's a nude Jacuzzi and steam room for women and you can do it before or after massage. Tons of people know about it here. Because I was training for the triathlon, I got a really strong knot in my neck and couldn't move it. So I went there for a chiropractor. But there's a hole in the wall I found called Bow Spa. There's no private room and it's maybe $45 for a whole hour of reflexology.

COVERING YOUR BASES

Of the major makeup categories, perhaps foundation has undergone the greatest transformation in recent years. Gone are the days when visible pancake was the default. Instead, women expect their foundation (or tinted moisturizers or BB creams—basically a tinted moisturizer pumped up with skin care benefits) to be seamless.

DIOR DIORSKIN FOREVER PERFECT MAKEUP with BROAD SPECTRUM 35

As a working mom, I have one chance a day to get my makeup on. This formula goes on easily, blends well, and is buildable for those less than stellar skin moments. But the loveliest surprise is this formula manages to have longevity without giving you "dead face"—a common problem with long-wearing formulas that go overboard on matte finishes.

MAC MATCHMASTER

Professional basketball player Skylar Diggins prefers this line for its inclusive color range. She tops off her application with a light dusting of matching MAC powder.

REN SATIN PERFECTION BB CREAM

For those after a natural look and feel—French fashion designer Julie de Libran likes this formulation because "it's light"—REN's BB cream is silicone-free.

GIORGIO ARMANI LUMINOUS SILK

This formula is likely in every celebrity makeup artist's kit and was widely considered a game changer when it was released. Why? Despite offering full coverage, it is also very lightweight and works well on HD cameras. As Juliette Lewis puts it: "Whoever discovered that formula must be really celebrating."

CHANEL PERFECTION LUMIÈRE VELVET

Nina Dobrev likes how this formula "covers well but not too much. Also, it has powder built into the foundation. It's great for someone on the go."

DIOR DIORSKIN AIRFLASH

Karla Souza reaches for this can when attending events. "It's a little cold when it comes out and it feels like there's a little mini de-puffing action happening," she says.

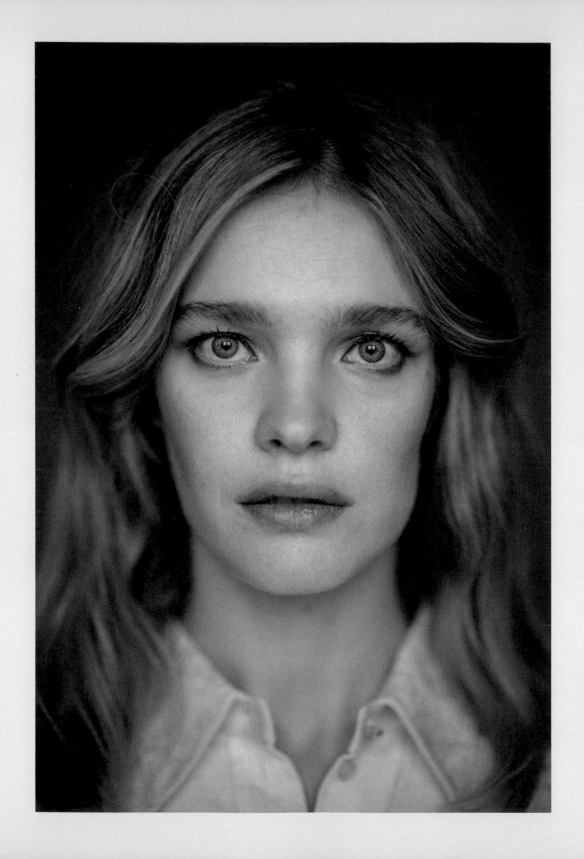

Natalia Vodianova

Model and Founder of

Naked Heart Foundation

SKIN CARE

The most important thing is to keep the skin clean and moisturized. Cleansing can be very rough on the skin, so I use a French pharmaceutical brand—La Roche-Posay—which is mild. Then for creams, I use the Super Aqua Day and Super Aqua Night creams by Guerlain. I'm an ambassador for the brand, but these are not the most famous products in the line. They are just ideal for me because I like how it's very smooth to put on makeup afterward.

Then, since I have very, very sensitive eyes, I use this cream that actually is a little pharmaceutical that my dermatologist recommended. It's called SVR Topialyse and it's specifically for irritated eyelids and anti-itching. It's not like my eyelids are itching all the time, but it's a really soft cream and it's soothing.

Another thing I'm absolutely loving is the Fresh Black Tea Firming Overnight Mask. Masks, the thing about them is that you have to put it on and leave it for a while and stay put and not do anything. It's really boring. I'm a mother; I don't have time for these things. The fact the mask is overnight is just a genius process. I pile it on and I go to bed and that's it. I don't have to think about it.

MAKEUP

I don't see much sun here in Paris, but I do still try to protect my skin. The BB cream from Guerlain has really good color and sun protection inside it. I do like a little bit of eye pencil during the day. Sometimes I don't even use mascara and just use the Charlotte Tilbury classic eyeliner powder pencil and maybe smudge it a tad. I also love Eyeko Brow Gel. The formula is not matte but has a little shine to it. My eyes are lighter and I think it's sometimes nice to have a darker brow to set them off. And I have these Fresh tinted lip moisturizers like Sugar Petal in my bag. They're so great because they're so easy.

One thing I learned from modeling is that a little shine in the corner of the eyes is really festive. You can use something shinier like Vaseline if you're really looking for light. But I like this beautiful Charlotte Tilbury pencil called Champagne Diamonds. It says it's for blue eyes—that's probably why I like it!

FRAGRANCE

During the day, I love the Calvin Klein Euphoria body lotion. It's so discreet but you feel fresh and extra clean somehow.

HAIR

My hair is very fine. I have a lot of it, especially right now—the whole pregnancy hair thing. But being a model, which means I undergo a lot of blow drying and a lot of pulling and different hair styles all the time when I work, it's important to rejuvenate the hair and to feed it as much as possible. I do a lot of Leonor Greyl. It's a very French brand and a hairstylist, Odile Gilbert, recommended it to me once. She said I should try the cream for the ends of my hair, so I went to look for it and discovered more. They have a little clinic in Paris and it's one of my only real indulgences because I'll go maybe every couple of weeks and it takes two hours, but you get a full head massage and amazing oils and masks. I feel like I had a week of holiday after I leave the place.

I also use a lot of Christophe Robin products at the moment. I get my hair colored by Christophe—I get it a little blonder than my natural color; I need the pick-me-up!—and I'll also get it cut at the salon when I'm there. I'm obsessed with his Volumizing Mist with Rose Water. And I do rotate shampoos, so when I'm not using Leonor Greyl, I like Christophe's Cleansing Milk with blueberry. It's really incredible.

OTHER SERVICES

I don't have time to pamper too much right now, but I do think it's an important thing for women to do. I'm actually looking for an acupuncturist in Paris. I have heard of a woman here, something-Wolf, and she's supposed to be incredible. But I need to get an introduction as she is apparently always booked up. Can you imagine how amazing she must be?

DIET AND FITNESS

What bothers me about yoga and Pilates is that I get very strong arms—very defined shoulders and such—very quickly. Everybody loves it, but I completely hate it. I don't want defined arms. I want to look very feminine. I want to have soft curves and not be too skinny and be in good shape but not to have defined arms. This always bothered me. Then I woke up one day and had, like, a revelation: "Ahh, I know what I want to do!" I'll do dancing because I figured, in dance, the arms are more like accessories.

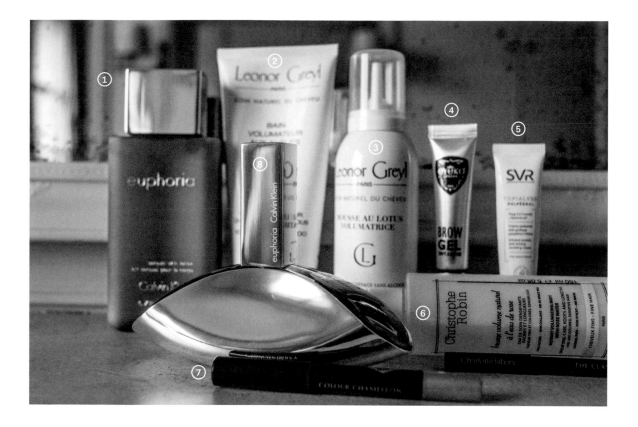

You never pull yourself up with your arms, but you do move them around. I found a lovely, very quiet dance studio where I take private classes. I do jazz and contemporary. I do it once a week, and there's something so wonderful about it. You get more in touch with yourself as a woman I think.

For diet, I do have rules. I follow the Blood Type Diet. I know a lot of people don't believe in it. But since I was a little girl, I've always had problems with my digestive system. I had ulcers, and then in my twenties, I was having really deep problems. Then I tried this, and in two weeks, I found a huge difference in how I felt. I'm lucky because I am AB blood type, I don't have to be too disciplined. I can still eat meat and carbs and fish. But there are rules, like I can't have red meat except for lamb. And same with vegetables—I can't have a ton of things but I'm allowed other things. I like it though. I've been doing it for more than ten years.

1 **Calvin Klein** Euphoria lotion

2 **Leonor Greyl** shampoo

3 **Leonor Greyl** Mousse au Lotus

4 **Eyeko** Brow Gel

5 **SVR** Topialyse Eye Cream

6 **Christophe Robin** Volumizing Mist with Rose Water

7 **Charlotte Tilbury** eye pencils

8 **Calvin Klein** Euphoria fragrance

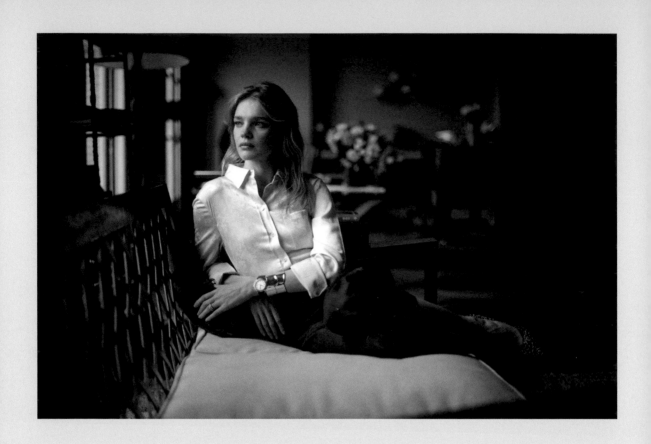

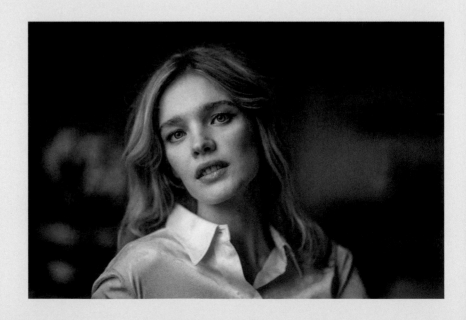

ALEXI LUBOMIRSKI
BEHIND the SCENES
of BEAUTY PHOTOGRAPHY

Though hair stylists and makeup artists influence an advertisement image or cover shot, walk onto any set and you'll quickly realize the photographer is running the show. I was familiar with Alexi Lubomirksi's work—he often shoots for publications and brands like *Allure*, *Vanity Fair*, Dior, and Lancôme—before we were seated next to each other at a Milk Makeup dinner. But whereas some photographers I've met think of their work purely in visual terms, it's refreshing that Alexi feels a responsibility for the kind of images he puts out there. (He admits he wasn't always this way. He became more aware after he became a father.) After all, an aspirational image often becomes a standard, however impossible to achieve. He cares enough that he even put out a book, called *Diverse Beauty*, in which he gives the cover-girl treatment to a variety of beauties. The idea? That aspiration can be manufactured and that a typical model face isn't the only covetable look around.

What happens on a beauty campaign shoot?
Usually the campaign comes from an ad agency. Before I even get there, they probably have come up with mountains of different ideas and ran them past the client and focus groups. When it finally comes to me, they might show me one idea or two ideas. One might be more out there, and one is the safer bet. I then give my input and try to do the one they dream of doing. After that, so many people are involved. There's the ad agency; there are the marketing teams who dissect whether this will work in certain countries. The way it works now, the industry is so global. You have to think about the different territories in the world, and they have different aesthetics and sometimes different religious beliefs.

But the truth is, if you're shooting advertising, you're an artist for hire. And you're a commercial artist. As much as you'd like to say, "It'd be amazing if we do this XYZ crazy spectacular look," at the end of the day, you have so many boxes to tick. These things cost millions of dollars to produce and then distribute. They have to play it safe.

The covers of magazines used to be much more creative. Now it's broken down to a science. If the hand is on the hip and the hair is down, you're going to sell more copies, or something like that. There are certain months though—those months that have less advertisers—where you can be more free.

Where is there still creativity?

Editorially, you can be much more fun. Even if you have to please an editor, it's more about selling a fantasy.

As a photographer, I try to make the experience, such as dealing with hair and makeup, collaborative. If it's advertising, they have tested everything up this point, so they'll say something like, "We're 90 percent sure we're doing the hair down." Of course, if that look truly doesn't work on a girl, then we are free to change it.

In editorial, it's much more of a discussion. I'll let hair and makeup know the idea or theme before the shoot so by the time we all get together at the beginning of the shoot, we can each offer some ideas. To me, there's no point in me telling them, "You're going to do this." They are the experts in their fields. It's important to remember it's not a dictatorship. It can be a balancing act though. As a photographer, you're like the host of the party, but you also don't want to stifle their creativity. You have to lead the horses but let them go in their particular field.

Do you think editorial images are still driving trends?

Oh it's totally driven by social media now. It's a brand-new crop of people—social media stars and bloggers. The dynamic has completely changed in the last five years. One of the last big campaigns I did, on one of the days I shot, they brought five to ten of the top beauty bloggers to watch and interview and record so they could immediately post their spin on the specific product or look as soon as the product comes out.

Before, the brands didn't have that option for behind the scenes. I'm sure people would have loved to see. As a photography student, I would have loved to watch the behind the scenes of a Helmut Newton shoot, for example. But it just wasn't that accessible. Today, when I get applications from a photography assistant, many didn't go to college for photography. Instead, they say they watched freeze frame YouTube videos to learn where the lights were.

On lights: How does makeup interact with photography? The makeup sometimes doesn't look good in real life. Sometimes on the set, people see the makeup and the girl. They say, "That looks crazy!" But as soon as the lights go on—and there are so many different types of light, the great makeup artists will know how to deal with each one—it might look stunning.

One change since the digital age: Makeup artists will put on a certain color palette and sometimes in the post-production process, the colors will completely morph. So I do try to work with the makeup artist very closely during postproduction. I want to make the shot have an emotional feel and feel like the color has not been compromised.

How does the image change in postproduction with tools like Photoshop?

The image does change. In the last eight years, people got very power crazy with the fact that you can retouch. The retouch arm is a long and twisted one. You have to be so responsible with what you are doing. Digital allows us to do more each day. For example, instead of doing five shots and getting each right, now it's, "Let's do ten shots and we'll fix these little things in postproduction."

On the other hand, it's important to keep the expression on the model's face. And if you rattle off ten shots, you're more likely to catch that expression before it dies. But the problem is: Who is policing this? Are you just taking out a pimple afterward or are you doing something to completely change the photograph? It can be a super fine line.

Do you think retouching has created aspirational but inaccessible images?

More and more you have to respect the intelligence of the viewer. With Instagram and beauty apps, people have retouching tools at their disposal. People now know that celebrities or models don't really look like that. So there's been less and less retouching on the extreme levels we've seen before. But there are ways to sell a fantasy and make it more approachable and relatable. So even though on the one hand it's great more are informed, on the other hand, there are still many who might look at these more "approachable" images and wonder how that particular subject could look that amazing.

When I think of postproduction Photoshop issues, they usually involve actresses—a group you often deal with. How has that been, working with celebrities?

It's been more and more about celebrities because now it's about the figures, numbers, and content a celebrity can bring. For example, if you're shooting for a magazine, and if you're shooting an actress who has a movie coming out, there's meat behind that story. If you're doing advertising and you're doing a celebrity, apart from the beautiful face, every time she comes out with a new movie or project, the brand will get another round of traction with the press.

You have to be sensitive as a photographer whether you're handling a model or a celebrity, but with models you are allowed more leeway. I can tell a model, "Do dancing cartwheels through Times Square wearing a tutu," and they'd say, "Great." With a celebrity, there's a whole new list of challenges you have to work around. Perhaps they want to represent themselves as a certain persona. Or maybe they don't want to be seen in a certain way. Maybe they have a serious movie coming out and they don't want to look too playful. Sometimes, they might have certain charities they're involved in that would conflict with the setup. Also, they have more insecurities. Like all of us, they have their flaws, and they are not eighteen-year-old models. As a photographer, you have to be gentler.

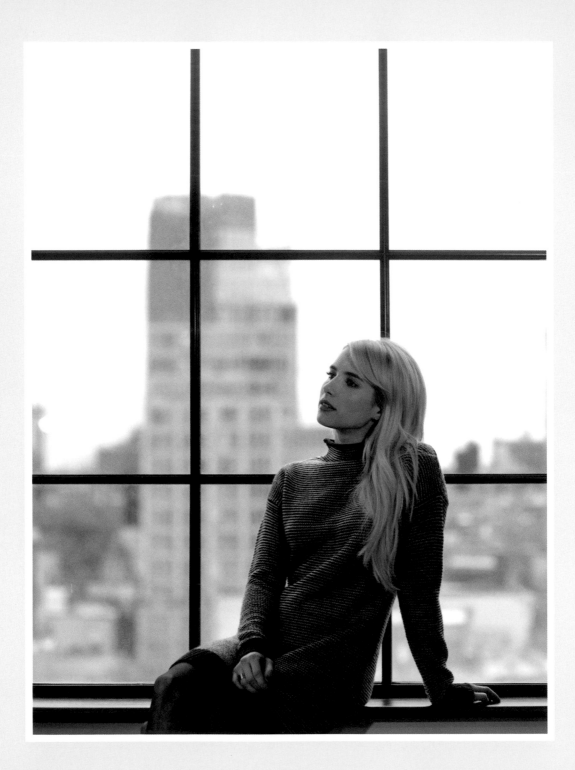

Emma Roberts

Actress

SKIN CARE

This is my favorite thing: It's my AmorePacific Dual Eye Creme and one is for day and one is for night. The day one has sunscreen in it. I believe it's new. I find out about products from reading. I am obsessed with beauty tips, and I'm obsessed with products. So I'm always reading online and magazines, and I'm always asking my friends what they are using. Also, we shoot in New Orleans, and on my days off I'll go to the Saks there and get new stuff. I love beauty counters.

Right now, I can't live without the Tata Harper Beautifying Face Oil. Then I use the Murad Oil-Control Mattifier SPF 15. It's great under makeup because the makeup goes really smoothly over it. I love the Neutrogena makeup remover wipes—I have literally ten packs of them. They're the only ones that don't make my eyes red.

Once a week, I love the REN Flash Rinse One Minute Facial—my friends recommended it to me. I have five of them because I'm always afraid things will get discontinued. Sometimes, I'll do the SK-II sheet mask. I've done those sheet masks in front of boyfriends before and scared the crap out of them. I don't get embarrassed in the name of beauty.

For my body, I just use almond oil I got from Whole Foods—I love the smell of it. If I'm showering in the morning, I dry brush. All the models always talk about it in articles, so I tried it out. I don't really see a visible difference but I do it anyway. I feel like it exfoliates a little bit.

MAKEUP

Some days when I'm not working, I might just do nothing. I'll just wear a pair of big sunglasses as my makeup. But otherwise, I'm not big on doing liner or shadow or a harsh lipstick during the day. On a day off, I'll use a little bit of an undereye concealer—I use Tom Ford—and Anastasia clear brow gel. I'll use a Shiseido eyelash curler and Chanel Inimitable mascara. I just started using the Honest Company Crème Blush—it's so pretty. And I can't live without the beautyblender sponge. If I'm wearing foundation, I like the Armani Luminous Silk one—Lea Michele told me about it. Then I just got this Bare Minerals Rose Passion lip color. It looks darker, but when you put it on, it's actually a little stain.

I'm always looking for great new colors, but I'm also good at throwing stuff out I don't use. Every two months, I'll throw out stuff out so there isn't an overflow. The only thing I hold on to is a good shade of red. So I have a lot of different red lipsticks at home. NARS does a really good one and so does Chanel.

FRAGRANCE

I love Le Labo Santal 33 and Neroli 36, because they don't smell perfume-y. I've become such a fan, I even bought their detergent. I wash my sheets in it. Also, I recently got the Miu Miu one and it's fun for going out at night. And the bottle is so cute—bottles matter.

HAIR

My natural color is dirty blonde. I either have to go blonde or brunette, otherwise it looks kind of mousy. I go to Nine Zero One salon in Los Angeles. Nikki Lee there does my hair and my extensions as do Riawna and Seama. Right now I have extensions for *Scream Queens*. When *Scream Queens* ends, I'm going to go and cut it all off. I love having it blonde and short because I can just roll out of bed and put some sea-salt spray in it and be out the door. I use Oribe's color-treated hair shampoo and I love their texture spray and hairspray. Sometimes, I'll do a Kérastase mask and I love the Serge Normant shine spray. That smells so good.

OTHER SERVICES

I just started doing acupuncture in New Orleans because the city is a really mystical place, and there are all these amazing, gifted people who are like healers almost. My acupuncturist's name is Quang, and he works out of his house, and he'll work on ten people at a time. I've noticed such a difference: It centers me and I feel like it gets the blood flowing. We work like twelve to fifteen hours a day, and you just get really drained.

I've also started getting cranial sacral massages. I have a serious jaw-clenching problem, and it's really helped with that. I go to this woman in the Bywater named Judy, and her cat lays on me while she massages. It's so fun!

Lately, I'm so into nail-polish. I love Julep. They do such good colors. I just got a blue that looks like denim. I don't do gel. I got gel a couple of times but when they filed them off, it really freaked me out. But when I get a day off in New Orleans, I love to get a coffee, go get my nails done,

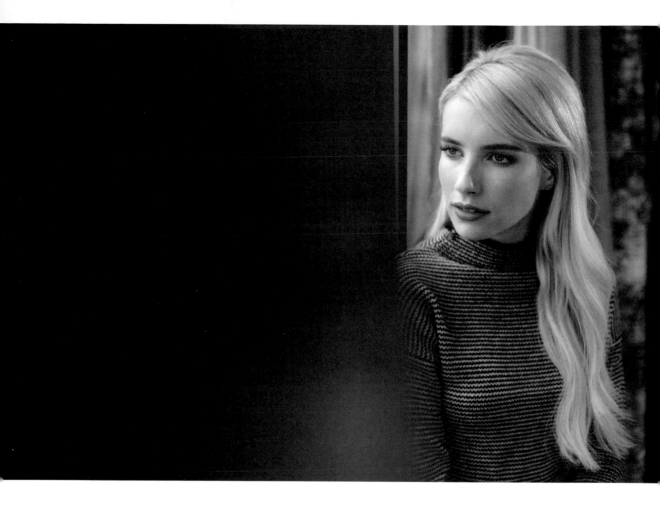

and go work out. I'm a total girly-girl in that sense.

DIET AND FITNESS

I'm about everything in moderation. I try to be healthy, but I will have dessert. We're shooting really long hours, so I always have Reese's Peanut Butter Cups and Swedish Fish on set because I have to have something to look forward to.

I'm not into gluten-free or any diets like that. I do try to vary what I'm eating though.

I am not a running person. Everyone laughs at me because my legs turn out when I run. I look absolutely ridiculous. I stopped running in seventh grade. But on our days off, Lea Michele—she's also in *Scream Queens*—and I will go do Pilates together. I also love yoga—I go to Reyn Studios in New Orleans. I like workouts that are good for your mind as well. With my job, your mind can get very noisy, and you can get a lot of anxiety. Sometimes I'll be up at night and not be able to sleep because I'll have anxiety about stuff. When I do Pilates and yoga, I'll sleep easier, and I'll feel a bit more that I can handle everything.

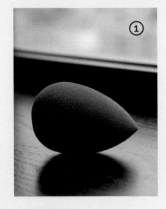

①

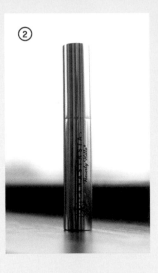

②

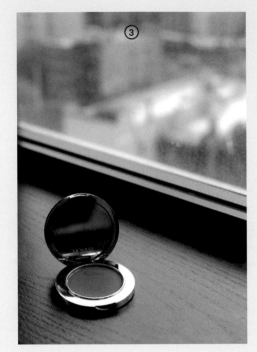

③

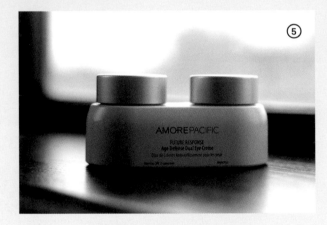

⑤

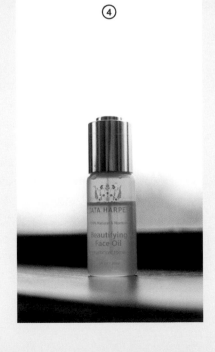

④

1   **beautyblender**
sponge

2   **Anastasia Beverly
Hills** Clear Brow Gel

3   **Honest Company**
Crème Blush

4   **Tata Harper**
Beautifying Face Oil

5   **AmorePacific**
Dual Eye Creme

AMY WECHSLER
THE PSYCHOLOGY OF WEARING MAKEUP TO WORK

Part and parcel of being a beauty editor is getting to know the best skin experts around. Case in point: I always learn something new when I speak with Amy Wechsler, M.D. She stands out for her dual board certifications: in dermatology and psychiatry. Considering how perceptions of beauty can affect the psyche, the double degree makes sense. But what has intrigued me since I started writing about beauty is how the topic can be perceived as frivolous vanity on the one hand but can seriously impact important issues on the other. I'm particularly thinking of several studies that have come out in recent years that conclude wearing some makeup in the workplace can increase promotions and overall success.

These studies, for me, all fall under the "attractive theory" that if you're more attractive you get more job offers and promotions. Our brains are wired to register, appreciate, and reward attractiveness. I don't love the double standard for women vs. men, but that is our culture.

Chanel also did these studies where subjects were shown different faces and asked to guess ages. All Chanel did was turn up or down the contrast on an image. When the contrast was increased, the subjects would think the person was prettier and younger. And that's what makeup does: It turns up the contrast on your face.

When I look at these studies, as a feminist, I really care how the woman feels about herself. If the only reason to wear makeup is that it's culturally demanded, that's not cool. On the other hand, for many women, wearing a little makeup is how they take care of themselves. Of course, this is also culturally informed. But if a woman puts on a little makeup and is well dressed and it helps with her self-confidence and posture, then it's good for her psyche. A little self-care can be a good and important thing.

Nicole Richie

Fashion Designer, Actress, and TV Personality

HAIR

I recently colored my hair. It's a lavender-slash-silver. My daughter asked me to do it, so I did. This change of color and all the maintenance is something new to me. Last July, I wanted to give my hair a break. I took all my extensions out for the first time in ten years and for seven months I was rocking only leave-in conditioner and a slick-back. I was giving my hair a chance to breathe because I do a lot to it. I color it and I do a Brazilian treatment. So I went from nothing to this color. It was a big jump.

With colored hair there are a lot of rules I'm learning. I just switched to this new natural shampoo by Davines and I use a color conditioner that my haircolorist Daniel Moon, who works at Andy Lecompte Salon, makes for me. He mixes up a combination of conditioner and color so that it deposits a little color each time.

Andy cuts my hair and has since I was nineteen. He's, coincidentally, one of my best friends. We're around the same age and started out, in a way, at the same time. Because I'm his friend, he can experiment with me. Every major haircut I've had is one that he's done. My attitude with beauty and hair is that it's temporary: You can always change it. It's how I feel about fashion as a whole as well. It's fun to see Andy and experiment and do it for over ten years. There's a history.

SKIN CARE

I take pretty good care of my skin. I use a lot of Dr. Lancer's products—he's someone I met

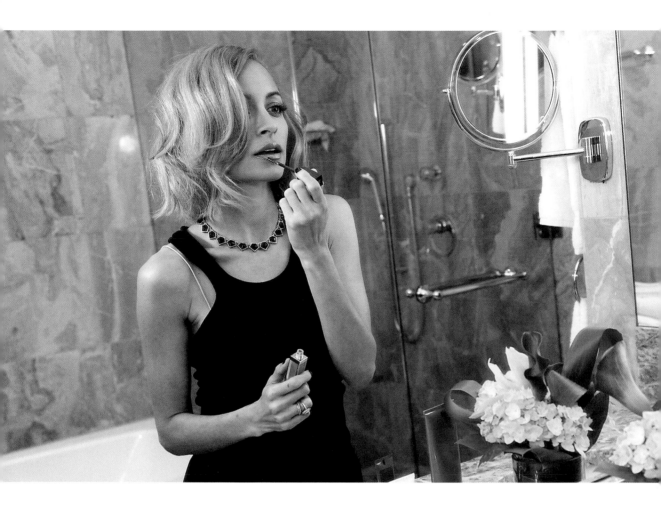

through my parents. I actually didn't see anybody until I was about twenty-three. I didn't know anything at all about skin care then. But I thought I should know more and my parents recommended him. He gave me the talk to stay out of the sun and gave me a few products as a preventive measure. Now, in the morning, I use his cleanser, polish, and moisturizer. That's it for my face. I don't use SPF. Dr. Lancer is on my case about it, but my parents told me "black don't crack."

At nighttime, it's pretty much the same routine, only I switch to a nighttime cream. To take makeup off, or if I'm traveling, I'll use the MAC cleansing wipes. I also have a bottle of makeup remover from Clinique.

MAKEUP

I don't wear a lot of makeup. I try, overall, to keep my skin hydrated and to let it breathe. I'll use Clé de Peau concealer to cover-up my undereye situation and CoverGirl mascara. Those are my go-tos. And I'll use a Shu Uemura eyelash curler to make my eyes more alive. I don't do a blush or a lip. I do use Lucas' Papaw

Ointment on my lips. I'll also stick it up my nose with a Q-tip when I fly, so I don't get sick. It works.

When I have an event, I work with a makeup artist. It's not something that I get to do in my everyday life, but it's fun to get dressed from head-to-toe. For me, it's not just about the clothes, it's also about hair and beauty. What is the overall look? How are you going to make a piece look different? I like to experiment. I think of it as a form of self-expression. I'm someone that is constantly testing herself and pushing her own boundaries. I could say I never wear blue eyeshadow, but then I've found myself in situations where that would work.

FRAGRANCE

I wear a combination of oils and lotion. My mother is Southern and very traditional and always taught me that you can't leave the house without smelling great and feeling great. Growing up, she would do oil in the shower and then get out and put on more lotions and oil. That's

something that has been passed down for sure. So in the shower, I have exfoliating gloves and I'll do soap—I like Dove—and then exfoliate with almond oil. When I get out of the shower, I combine a little grapeseed oil with the Kiehl's Creme de Corps with Soy Milk and Honey, which has a light scent to it. When I'm dry—I tend to be a little on the dry side—I'll use CeraVe. After that, I have different perfume oils, like muguet. I'll pick them up anywhere or my mom will send over oils. She travels a lot. Then, I'll spray on my perfume over that. I probably smell a little different every day.

SERVICES

Kimmie Kyees does my nails. Nail art is a little aggressive for me. I did a version of it, a very toned down version, for the Met Ball last year and that was fun and safe. But I pretty much stick to nudes, reds, and blacks. Same goes for toes.

I don't get facials and I'm extremely ticklish. I'm one of the few people who hate

massages. I just cannot do them. I also don't like the idea of being stuck in a room with somebody.

FITNESS

I go to Tracy Anderson. I've been working with her over three years now. She's wonderful. She's small like me and she knows my body type and is very on point with that whole world.

DIET

As far as diet, we don't diet here. But I'm very conscious of what my family eats. We grow a lot of our own fruits and vegetables at our house. Currently we are growing kale, spinach, broccoli, three kinds of tomato, arugula, and we grow all of our own herbs as well. I hope to be a green thumb. If you make that the standard for the family, it becomes habit. But my whole thing is that you have to enjoy yourself too. We eat healthy and clean, but of course there are times when you got to "wile out."

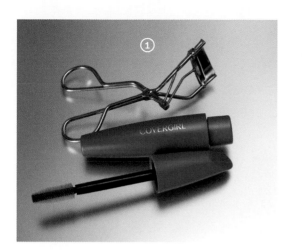

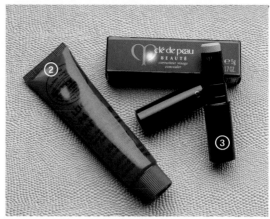

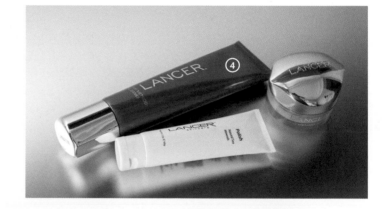

1 **CoverGirl**
mascara

2 **Lucas' Papaw**
Ointment

3 **Clé de Peau**
concealer

4 **Lancer The Method:**
Cleanser, Polish,
Moisturizer

5 **Davines**
shampoo

6 **Kiehl's**
Creme de Corps with
Soy Milk and Honey

7 **Body Time**
Muguet perfume oil

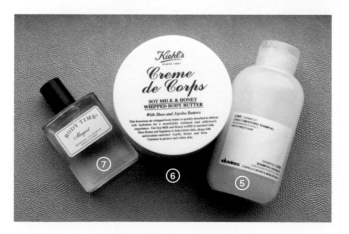

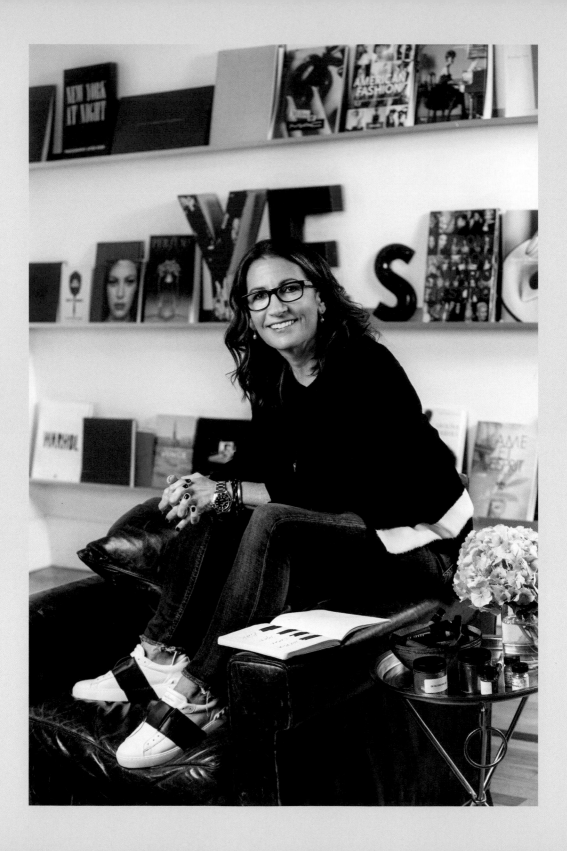

Bobbi Brown

Founder, Bobbi Brown Cosmetics

SKIN CARE

I don't cleanse my skin in the morning because I cleanse it so perfectly at night. I just splash water on it. And I'll sometimes use the Extra Treatment Lotion. It looks like a toner but it's not. It actually has some moisture to it. And I wear SPF 25 and moisturizer every day. I have super dry skin. My skin care routine in the morning is about hydration. One of the things I do is I go down to the kitchen and drink two glasses of water. Now I'm doing warm water because my Indian doctor told me it's better for your digestion.

Things change at night. Certainly as you get older, things change. You get drier. So I layer. I start with my Extra Repair Moisturizing Balm. It's densely moisturizing. If you took away my entire line and said you could have one thing, that would be the one thing I'd keep—above the makeup. Makeup is on your skin but if your skin isn't hydrated, it doesn't look good. For really, really dry days, I put my face oil on top of that. I've had a face oil for probably fifteen years. It has neroli in it, so my husband loves the way it smells.

I do masks about once a week. I leave them in my shower. Someone told me to do that as a tip. Before I go in the shower, I put it on. I'm not one of these fluffy people who actually takes care of myself as well as I should when I'm home. But this season, I'm traveling a bunch. I'll bring a mask with me to do in the hotel. I also bring those teeth whitening things with me. I'm trying the Dr. Apa one—it's fancy. I'm still figuring out if it works.

MAKEUP

When I'm in the office and having product development meetings, I don't know what I look like. I try everything. We have a new line of lipstick coming out, and I literally tried every single one because I wanted to make sure there was enough color in it when you put it on your lips—it's a very special formula. Then I tried this gel liner that I didn't love, but then I smudged it and made it into a smoky eye, which I did love. Then I put some shimmery glittery things on top of it. Thank god I went out with friends last night because I looked like a mess.

Or a rock star! I looked like a rock star, that's it.

For my day to day, it's that kind of makeup where you can't tell you're wearing a lot. I wear Tinted Moisturizing Balm often. I've been playing with the new retouching wands we have. It was a really bad concealer formula that we poured into this cool thing with a wand, and it dispersed it so sheer, it made it look like you were retouched. I call it the Cinderella wand for your face, but I couldn't call it Cinderella, clearly—someone already owns it. I'll do color-correcting with my products but I don't do it with those colors. I don't do green or purple anything. It just makes you look like you have green and purple on.

I usually do bronzer, either Telluride or Stonestreet and Elvis Duran, which were made for two men I know: Eric Stonestreet of *Modern Family* for the first one and Elvis. I do throw a blush on top of that—just a little pink. And I do mascara. When I get around to doing my eyebrows, that makes me really happy.

It really does make a difference. But I don't know about eyebrow trends.

I don't think anyone looks good with runway makeup in real life. The unibrow? Very cool on the Gucci runway or whatever show. Walking down Broadway in Soho? A little scary. But I've never been a big trend person when it comes to makeup. I'd much rather do trends on my feet or my jewelry. Makeup I always like just pretty and subtle.

At night, I'll throw a highlighter on over my bronzer and blush. But what you'll never see me in is a red lip. You'll never see me in a dark vampy lip either, because I don't look good in it. I do lippy colors. I have one color called Bobbi. It's kind of a purple-y nude color that I wish my lips were because I don't really like the look of lipstick on me.

HAIR

Today, I have a blowout. I go to Marissa from Marie Robinson. She does my cuts too. I've been going to her for two years. I go to a salon

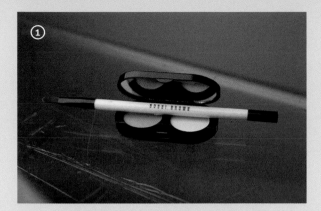

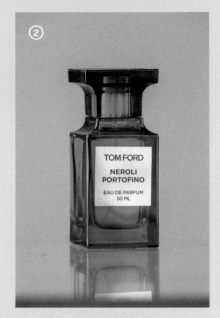

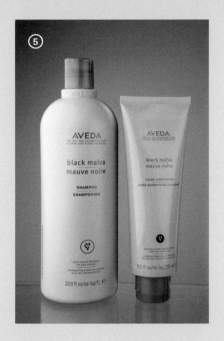

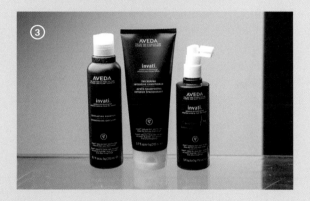

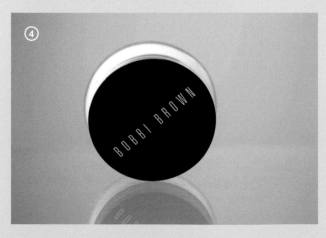

1 **Bobbi Brown** Tinted Moisturizing Balm

2 **Tom Ford** Neroli Portofino

3 **Aveda** Invati

4 **Bobbi Brown** Extra Moisturizing Balm

5 **Aveda** Black Malva Shampoo, Color Conditioner

in New Jersey—I'm based in Montclair—for color, though, because I get it colored so often. My hair is white. I've been white since I was twenty-five. My dad has beautiful white hair. I've worked really hard on making sure my hair doesn't look orange or red because I like normal hair color. There are highlights in there now but I'm getting rid of them tomorrow. And you can't tell that I have white roots because I have eye shadow in my part. My hair grows really fast. I use either my Mahogany or Espresso shadow with a damp brush, which is great because when you travel you can do the little parts. Sometimes, I also use the Sepia Ink eye gel with a little brush that I've destroyed. It can be tricky though. The shadow is easier.

Mahogany, for me, is my part, my eyebrows, my eyeliner. I can smudge it, and guess what, I once used it on lips because my assistant forgot the lip palette and I had to think quickly. It was for Rachel Roy's fashion show, and she wanted dark lips. I took balm and the Mahogany and it was written about in *Vogue.* Good things can happen out of disasters.

For shampoo and conditioners, I have so many things. I switch off so much. I've used Bumble and bumble, and I love the Aveda Black Malva—the smell lingers nicely.

FRAGRANCE

All my fragrances have to start with Bs. And all my kids have Ds. Some people call me "Rain Man." We have a fragrance oil called Bed that has neroli and patchouli in it. I called it Bed because whenever I put it on, that's where my husband wants to go. We didn't ever really do anything with it when we launched it though. Then people started asking about it, so we brought it back. But for me, I dabble in so many different fragrances and brands. I love some of the indie things and some of the oils. Padma Lakshmi, I was at a party with her and I was like "You smell so good." She said, "I make this special perfume." She gave it to me, and I wear it a lot. I think there's definitely neroli and patchouli. I generally like fresh showery things but neroli and patchouli is always good. Tom Ford has a great one.

I'm also addicted to this peppermint oil by EO. You use it on your hands. But in a pinch, it smells really good on the skin. Every single artist of mine has this with them. It feels fresh, especially if you're sweaty at the end of the day.

OTHER SERVICES

I do everything and am open to anything. I do a lot of holistic things. My second son is actually dating an acupuncturist. The other night, she did me.

With my Indian doctor, Amy Shah, it's all online. I met her on Instagram. She's amazing. She's 100 percent helped my digestion through diet recommendations and a supplement she suggested. The way we met, she saw a picture I posted—a picture with all these digestive things—when I was in Italy, and she reached out and said, "I can help." I actually knew of her already, because I watch a lot of those mindbodygreen classes. I want to go back to school to learn about these things. I had bought her class before.

Also, we have a manicurist who's here every day in the office doing manicures for everybody. Often she'll be in the room during meetings. If you're a mom and you're in the beauty business, you've got to have a manicure and this saves time. I do essie Geranium in the summer. And this is Berry Naughty I have on now.

DIET AND FITNESS

I go to a place called Parabolic, which is strength and conditioning. There are five to seven people at a time with like three trainers. Everyone has their own programs but the trainers are there to help. If you do hurt yourself, you also have physical therapists and acupuncturists there. I used to do spin—I used to do everything—and I kept hurting myself. I've never had better posture and never felt stronger since I've gone there. It's a lot of balance work, which is really important as you get older. They also teach you breathing, which no one

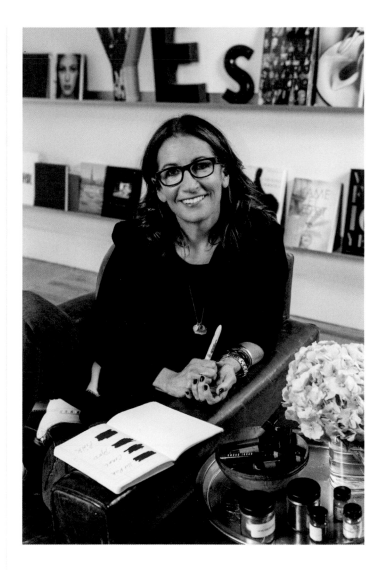

ever teaches you. Breathing changes everything. And I walk five to seven days a week between 10,000 to 20,000 steps a day. On weekends— the kids are out of the house now—my husband and I walk the entire day.

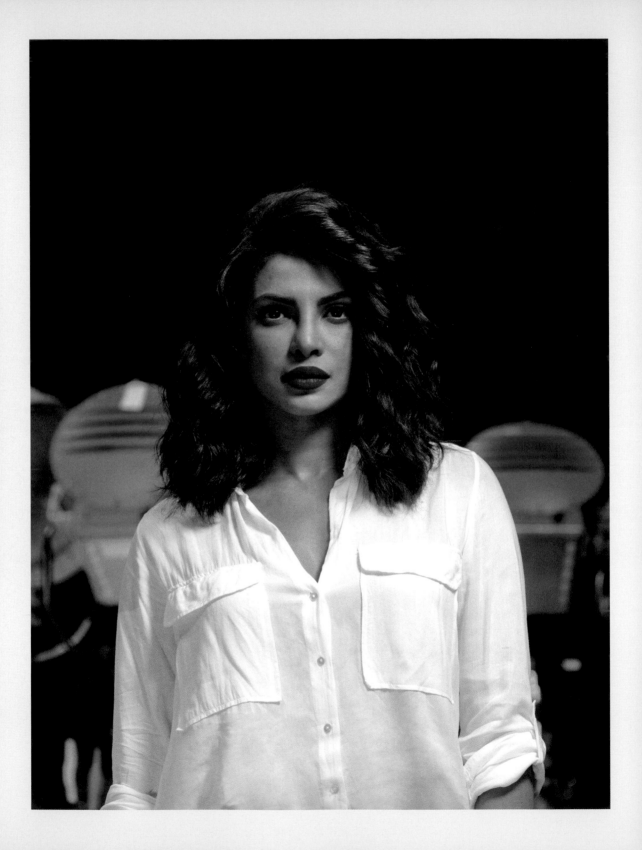

Priyanka Chopra

Actress

MAKEUP

I'm in the makeup chair almost every day. It's an interesting thing, the concept of "beauty" as an actor. People have doubted my abilities because of my beauty, and I've enjoyed proving to them that beauty shouldn't have anything to do with your ability to tell the story. It's important for actors to be chameleons. Beauty is just one aspect.

If I'm not working, I use the Armani foundation under my eyes if I need to. Then it's mostly just lip balm or a lip stain. I like the lip stains by Laura Mercier. I also like the MAC and NARS lipsticks when I'm doing something bold. For MAC, I have Lady Danger, Candy Yum-Yum, Ruby Woo, Russian Red, and Studded Kiss. NARS, I like the Dolce Vita. I stick with the matte lipsticks. I don't wear gloss. I have really big lips, and when I wear gloss they look way bigger. I have to keep them in check!

My mom wears kohl all the time. It's an amazing look and part of our culture for eons. Kohl makes big brown or black eyes stand out that much more. But I'm not big on the smoky eye. I like to keep the eye fresh.

I just use YSL mascara and then an Anastasia Beverly Hills pencil for my brows. I actually use my fingers to curl up my mascara. I'm not very meticulous when it comes to my makeup. I pretty much use my fingers, except I'll use a brush for my blush. Right now, I'm using a Chanel powder blush in Rose Ecrin. The color comes off very natural.

SKIN CARE

What is most important for your skin care is what you do the night before. You have to remove all remnants of makeup before you go to bed no matter how tired you are. And then, of course, you have to moisturize and cleanse. I double wash because I wear a lot of makeup when I work. Right now, I'm using the Chanel Intense Brightening Foam Cleanser followed by the MAC Green Gel Cleanser. I have dry skin, but it's still very important to take off all the makeup and grime. I also double moisturize. I use the Kiehl's serum called Daily Reviving Concentrate and then a cream by Tatcha. I've also found that StriVectin undereye cream really works for me. I am also trying some lip balms by StriVectin right now. For my body, I moisturize with Bio-Oil and a body lotion from Diptyque. If I'm going in the sun, I wear a face sunscreen by Shiseido. I find most of my products from reading magazines and also listening to what makeup artists tell me to do. And I usually do all my shopping at the duty-free, so I keep trying new things and find out what works.

Whenever I'm tired or getting on a flight, I'll wear the SK-II mask. I'm usually in a cabin on the plane, and I just shut the door and put it on. Or sometimes if I have the time, I'll put on fresh yogurt as a mask with a little turmeric powder in it—this is like an Indian trick. The turmeric is a healer for your skin.

FRAGRANCE

It's very important to me. It makes me feel like I'm walking around in my own bubble. Right now I'm using Dolce & Gabbana The One and Diptyque L'Ombre dans l'Eau. I'm a big fan of Diptyque, which I discovered at duty-free. I travel so much, my beauty information comes from there!

HAIR

I'm very blessed with Indian genes. I have good hair. When I was young, my grandmother used to give me coconut oil head massages. I used to say, "I don't want it!" but now of course I know how great it was. I like Oribe products. I love the smell and I find the products make my hair glossy. I use the shampoo, conditioner, and maybe a serum. Because I'm sitting in the hair and makeup chair all the time, my hair gets blown out, but my hair is actually wavy. I let it be and pull it back if it's my day off. For haircuts, I get trims. I can't change it much because I'm always filming some scene for a character and you need continuity. I'm telling a story.

OTHER SERVICES

I try to get massages whenever I can, but I'm not very fussy. I go to a nice spa in the city I'm in, or I go for a massage at home—somebody that does house calls.

DIET AND FITNESS

You're going to be very bored with this answer, but I don't do anything for fitness. I realize it's my genes and my age. I'm going to take advantage of it as long as I can!

For diet, hydration is very important. I drink a lot of coconut water. They have electrolytes, which are good for you. And especially in Mumbai, the coconuts are so fresh.

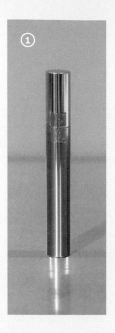

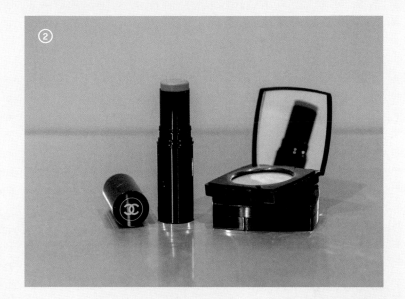

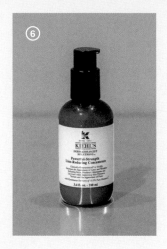

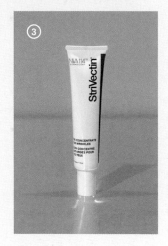

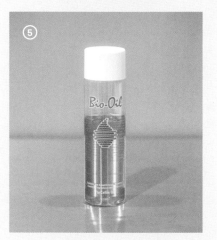

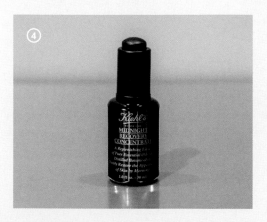

1 Yves Saint Laurent
mascara

2 Chanel
Powder Blush in Rose
Ecrin, Cream Blush

3 StriVectin
undereye cream

4 Kiehl's
Midnight Recovery
Concentrate

5 Bio-Oil

6 Kiehl's
Powerful-Strength
Line-Reducing
Concentrate

KIRA NASRAT
HOW TO DO BOLD, BELIEVABLE BROWS

Kira Nasrat's work isn't the kind that screams for attention, but when I spot a well-balanced look on the red carpet, chances are I'll look up the artist and she's the one wielding the makeup brushes. I especially associate her style with her client Jessica Alba, who represents an approach-able pretty that many women aspire to. One example of her skill: Kira is able to translate the bold brow trend in a way that's obvious yet not overwhelming.

Bold brows, they come and they go. Unfortunately, once they're gone, and you keep them gone for a really long time, sometimes they tend to not resurface. I'm talking about the '90s and the Drew Barrymore pencil-thin brow. I know a lot of people who still have not recovered from that era. Right now, the current brow is more of an '80s thing. That decade, there was more of a feathery brow going on. I think of Brooke Shields.

For today's brow, it's important to keep in mind that no matter what trend is going on, you should maintain your brows according to your face. That's something people tend to ignore. Not all brows are created equal. They come in different shapes and colors. You have to really embrace your shape and not overtweeze.

The thing about the super strong brows you see—a lot of people have called them Instagram brows or reality brows—they might not suit your face. Your face is the artwork; your brows are the frame. So you really have to understand the architectural positioning of where everything—your eyes, your nose, etc.—falls in relation to your brows.

TIPS FOR THE BEST FULL BROWS

First, you can totally have fun with your brows, but know that if you tweeze them, there's a consequence. If you want a fuller look, you should probably just clean up your natural shape. What I do is I brush up the brow hairs and see how they look. Then you just trim a little bit here and there and tweeze only the excessive hairs.

If you're filling in your brows, don't go too dark when choosing the color. If you go too dark, they can overpower your face. Even if your hair is naturally black, you want to use a dark brown pencil. Redheads, it's prettier to not match your pencil to your hair identically, but to find a shade that has a warmth to it, like a brown-red pencil. Blondes, don't go too brown if you're naturally blonde. But if you have darker roots, it's ok to go with a darker brow.

When filling in, I prefer to use a fine pencil with some wax to it. I draw in little fine lines. If you need it, you can combine the pencil with a little bit of powder applied with a slanted brush. Or if you have more brow, you can do a colored brow gel.

One of the most common mistakes I see is overfilling your brow. If you overfill, they can obscure your eyes. A good test for brow shape is to step back and ask yourself: Do your brows make your eyes pop? The right brows will make the eyes stand out.

If you don't have much brow hair, I always suggest trying eyebrow serum. But if you're trying to draw in a brow from very little hair, I start off with a lighter color to create the shape first. Then I go back with a darker shade to draw in little hairs. It comes off more believable that way.

One application tip: When I'm prepping a client's face, I'll put moisturizer all over but I'll skip the brows. If you need to go to an event or are prone to wandering brows, then you can also put oil-free primer in the brow area. This helps everything go on smoothly and stick.

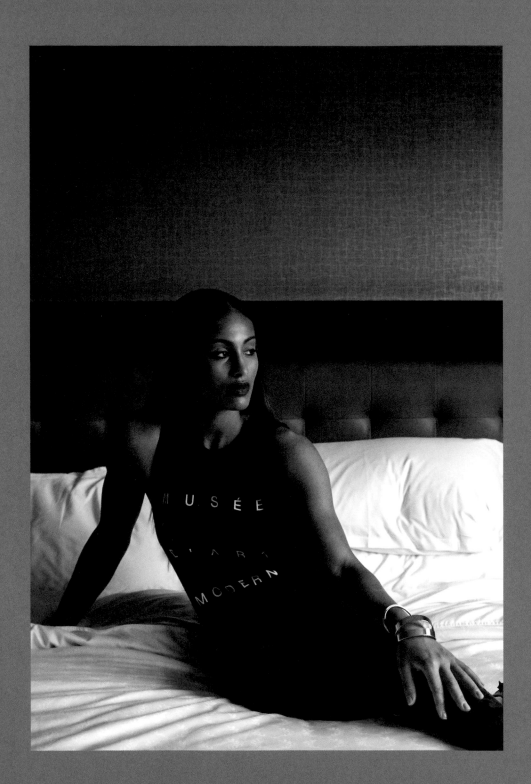

Skylar Diggins

Basketball Player

SKIN CARE

When in season, I wake up at about 7:30 every day, have breakfast, and try to get to the gym by 8:30 A.M. Before I'm out the door, I have to have a shower. I'm OCD with my showers. You have to be diligent with showering, with how much you sweat. On game days, I'll shower four times. It's so weird. Anyway, I like Tone scented shower gel. I love the Mango Splash with cocoa butter and the blue one, which is Ocean Therapy. After, I'll use Palmer's cocoa butter lotion all over and then Dove deodorant.

I switch up my facial wash. Right now, I like Simple Moisturizing Facial Wash. Simple has a great moisturizer too. I grab it from a CVS store. Some days, I'll just use a Dove bar. For me, products are really trial and error. Everyone is different, and to each her own as far as what works. They don't have to be the most expensive products. I've tried products on both ends of the spectrum and I just use what I like.

When I'm traveling, I always have face wipes in my bag. I like the Neutrogena makeup remover ones that work on mascara, which can be a pain to take off. For lips, I like eos lip balm in a fruit punch–type flavor. It looks like an egg. I also use a beeswax lip balm that comes in a yellow tube.

MAKEUP

All of my makeup is MAC. I've tried different brands, but with the colors, I just ended up sticking with MAC. During the day, I might use a little liquid Matchmaster foundation with a little powder. Then I use Skinfinish—I love the bronzed look it gives you—a little mascara and lip gloss and I'm out the door.

The only thing I change when I'm going out at night is the lip. I'll do pinks or a matte red. My go-to is Rihanna's RiRi Woo color.

FRAGRANCE

I love the Victoria's Secret Bombshell Diamonds scent, and in the past I've used Dolce & Gabbana Light Blue. It's light. But with fragrance, I think it can be overkill. I rely more on my scented lotions. I love the Victoria's Secret lotion that goes with the perfume—it has a bit of sparkle to it. Also, I have the Bath and Body Works body creams. I'm pretty much into anything with a fruity smell—I can't handle the spicy scents—like mangos tend to be my favorite. I feel like I've had them all.

HAIR

Changing up my hair is my thing. I don't wash it every day, but I definitely try to keep it conditioned. I'll use anything with argan oil, and I'll go out and buy the little travel tubes for when I'm on the road. You don't want to rely on the hotel stuff.

I have a lady in South Bend that does my hair when I go home. I also have three or four stylists that I stick to that will travel to Tulsa. I definitely straighten my hair—my natural hair has a very curly pattern. You know how it goes: Everyone who has curly hair wants straight hair and likewise. And I also get extensions. Currently, it's

like an ombré. I've had ombré where it's been really light and then also a honey color; I've had an ombré that went into plum. I try to change it up each time. I play with the lengths too. With extensions, I find it's better for your hair when you can play with color and length without damaging your hair.

Depending on how often I'm washing my hair, I might be changing my hairstyle every few weeks. I like to mix it up and explore. Sometimes I'll go back and look at photos and look at my hair and be like "What was I thinking?" It's like a period of time in your life. But I wasn't always like this. I was pretty much a ponytail athlete for most of my life. Then, after going to college, I started experimenting with different styles off the court. I'm an athlete, but at the same time I love my femininity.

OTHER SERVICES

I get manis, pedis, massages, all of the above. I try to get a mani once a week. I tend to do nude natural colors, especially

if I have a stretch of photo shoots. And being on my feet a lot, I try to do the same with my pedicure, but I'll play with more brights. In my work, you get stepped on and it's start and stop; it's really harsh movement and hard on your feet. Besides, it's now sandal weather. It warrants immediate pedi attention.

DIET AND FITNESS

Part of fitness is my job, but the other part is that it's my responsibility for taking care of my body. If I'm not on the court, I do high-intensity training, intervals, functional movement, strength, and core. And I have to eat clean: a lot of greens, fish, and chicken. I don't eat a ton of red meat. I do allow myself cheat meals. But people will ask about how to stay in shape, and it's all about diet. That and sleep. I'll nap between my shoot-around and game time. And I try to get six to eight hours every night.

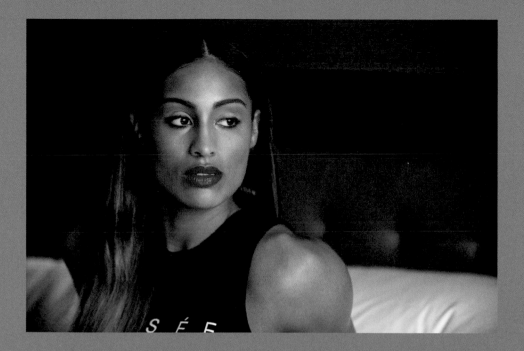

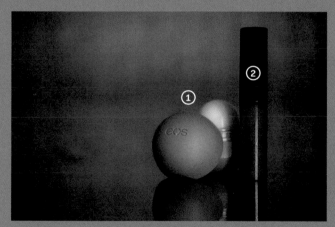

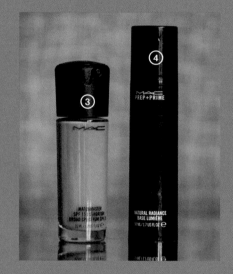

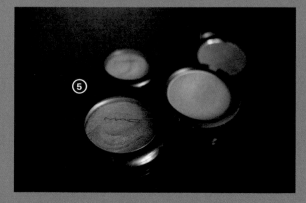

1   **eos** lip balm

2   **MAC** lip gloss

3   **MAC** Matchmaster Foundation

4   **MAC** Prep + Prime Natural Radiance Base Lumiére

5   **MAC** Skinfinish

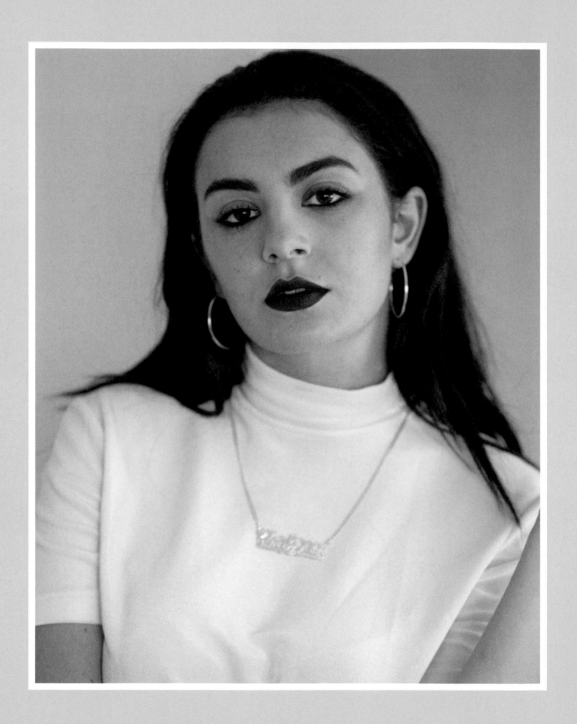

Charli XCX

Musician

MAKEUP

To be honest, my usual makeup is the same as in my music video looks. I really like doing a matte red lip and black around my eyes, with this clear gloss from MAC I'll use on my lids and kind of on the brow bone. The red I always use is NARS Cruella. When I was younger, I was quite scared of a red lip. But then I started listening to French '60s Yé-yé pop when I was making *Sucker*. I was looking at Brigitte Bardot and those kind of girls. When they were dressed up, it was often a bold red lip.

I think big brows are pretty cool. Yeah, I'll color them in a little bit. I use the Anastasia Beverly Hills brow pencil. But this dark shade is super natural. When I was growing up, I kind of rocked the Frida Kahlo quite a lot.

I really like the Rimmel ScandalEyes Mascara. It's simple and easy to just load on and still look nice and give a really bold lash. It's also really easy to buy. I can buy it in any country, which

is awesome. Then I'll use this Burberry kohl eyeliner on my water line and smudge it on my edge as well. They also do a liquid eyeliner. When I was younger, I was obsessed with how to do a liquid line. That's the one thing I'm good at when it comes to makeup.

And my makeup artist introduced me to Armani Luminous Silk Foundation. It doesn't ever look thick.

It's pretty much the same at night. Maybe I'll add more black around my eyes. Or do a different kind of lip, like a fuchsia. Or it's an idea: I think about the '90s. I'm a really big fan of movies like *Clueless* and *Jawbreaker*. For example, at the VMAs, we did white eye shadow and baby pink lips. It was dreamy and girly—a Cher Horowitz vibe.

SKIN CARE

In the morning, I just wash my face with Kiehl's. It's the one that comes in a blue bottle and it's an oil-free cleanser. I'll do that in the shower. After I get out, I'll use the blue liquid Kiehl's toner that goes with it. I have this super nice Chanel moisturizer—it smells really nice; it's kind of fresh—and I'll put that all over. I discovered it from doing a lot of photo shoots. And also it's got a really glamorous look, and I just wanted to have that in my box.

But I get kind of lazy when I'm on tour. It's a lot of face wipes—I like Johnson's. It's made for babies, but that's what my mom used to buy for the home. My mom is terrible with makeup—so no words of wisdom there—but the one thing she does tell me is to drink loads of water. I also use rose water. That freshens me up as well. I started doing that at South by Southwest two years ago. I found it in a dressing room. The one I've been using is from Urban Outfitters.

FRAGRANCE

I really like Daisy by Marc Jacobs—the "fresh" one with the multicolored flowers on top. I'm a really visual person, so I always pick the bottles that look the best. I also like the Burberry Brit fragrance. And I actually love a lot of Victoria's Secret body sprays. They're not super strong. They kind of make me feel like a princess when I wear them.

HAIR

My hair is naturally super curly. But I really don't do so much to it. I never brush it that much. I just sleep on it and see what happens. In the shower, I'll use Bumble and bumble shampoo and conditioner—the one for dry hair. My hair is often under irons and things. I don't get my hair cut. I never book an appointment. Sometimes people will cut it when I'm on shoots and that's about it. One product I'll always use and stand by: After Party by this company called TIGI. It's an amazing bottle that looks like a dildo. And it smells great. I'll put some on after I wake up and it'll smooth things out.

Sometimes I'll dye my hair darker when I'm feeling gothic, but my hair has always been dark brown. When I was younger, I wanted to be blonde because Baby Spice was blonde. But right now I'm feeling brown. I do like wigs too. I just bought a ton of wigs from Claire's Accessories and one is neon pink.

SERVICES

There's a place in New York called Valley that is really good for nails. A friend of mine, who has blue hair and great nails, said to go there. I was actually asking her where to go to get a wax, and she goes, "You *have* to go to Valley." Nails and wax in one go. I don't get nail art because I'm scruffy and messy and it always falls off. I like it plain with just one color. I really like the Chanel polishes, like in Rouge Noir or Pirate.

DIET AND FITNESS

I don't think about either really. Never. But generally going on stage an hour a night is enough for me. Someday, I will probably have to. I'm young, but I also love fried chicken.

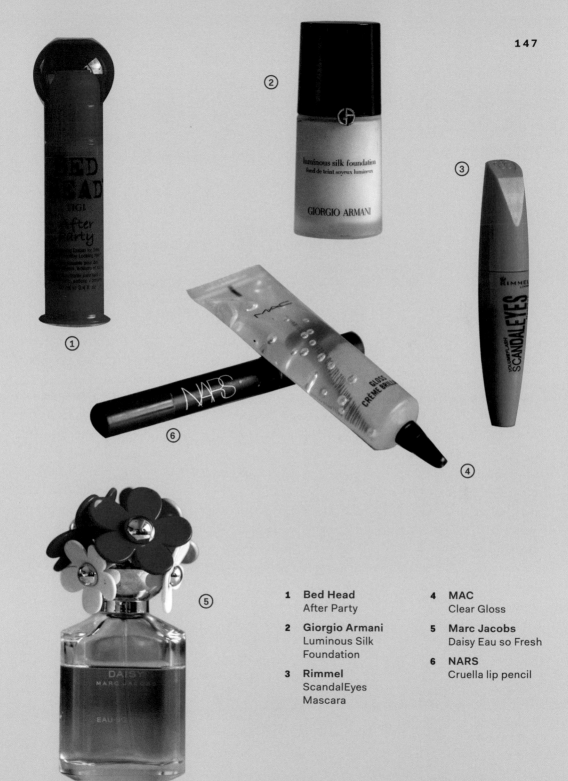

1   **Bed Head**
After Party

2   **Giorgio Armani**
Luminous Silk
Foundation

3   **Rimmel**
ScandalEyes
Mascara

4   **MAC**
Clear Gloss

5   **Marc Jacobs**
Daisy Eau so Fresh

6   **NARS**
Cruella lip pencil

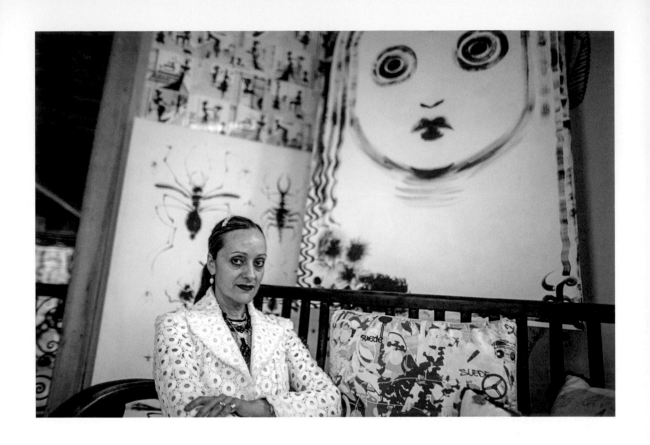

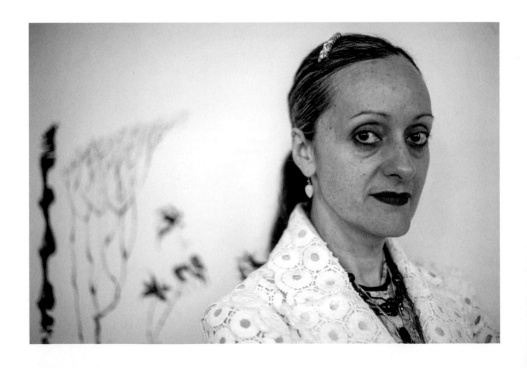

Isabel Toledo

Fashion Designer

FRAGRANCE

I use different scents at one time. I call them my North and South scents. For North, which is what I dab around the crown of my head and my hair, I use Gardénia by Chanel. Ruben, my husband, bought it for me a long time ago, and I've been using it for years. My South scent, which is what I put in the valley and mountains, is very special. It's Frédéric Malle Carnal Flower, and the scent comes up from your cleavage only every so often, especially if you get hot all of a sudden. Then you'll get just the most beautiful whiff.

SKIN CARE

I have Maja soap bars, which come from Spain. I've been using them since I was a kid, and it's the brand my mother used and my grandmother. I also keep SK-II face wash in the shower and I'll cleanse with that. Then after I'm done, but while my skin is still wet, I'll put on Johnson's baby oil all over. It really leaves your skin nice and moisturized. I might, on dry days, also use a bit of Car-ita Fluide de Beauté 14, which I dab on both my hair and skin. And I love a good hand cream. It's a necessity when you work with your hands—I don't want to snag a gorgeous fabric with brittle nails or skin. I use La Mer hand cream or one by Dr. Hauschka.

After, I use Chanel Sublimage for my face moisturizer. I discovered it at a photo shoot. Somebody used it on me, and it felt very silky and I thought, "I must have this." It is an expensive treat, but I use it sparingly and it goes a long way. I don't use sunscreen, funny enough, and I don't use eye cream. I think the moisturizer is enough. Sometimes at night, which is basically the same routine, I'll also use the Estée Lauder Advanced Night Repair and let that soak in while I dream. And, if I have been out on the town, I use Klorane to remove makeup. It's very gentle, almost like rainwater.

MAKEUP

I was born with red lips! When I was younger, I used to also wear some oranges and corals, but once I got to a certain age, I just kept the red. It's almost a uniform now, and it just makes you look sexy. I wear Chanel Rouge Allure red lipstick in 99 - Pirate every day, and you'd be surprised how many shades you can get with just one color. Usually, during the day, I just dab it on. Then I'll do black eyeliner pencil and sometimes I'll smudge it on. I particularly like MAC's pencil in Smolder. Then I'll dust on some Maja powder, which was also something my mother used. Maybe it's psychological at this point, because I kind of react to the scent of it.

At night, my look is the same, but I have a heck of lot more on. I'll really put on the red lipstick. I wear Shiseido powder foundation, and I'll keep a Chanel compact in my purse. I also use Lancôme Hypnôse mascara. I might wear a smoky shadow with a bit of unexpected color. It's beautiful to have maybe just a little green liner on the lash line. MAC has a great assortment of colors, like an artist's palette. Beauty is connecting your looks to your feelings. I like to use makeup to surprise and inspire myself with a bit of fantasy.

HAIR

In the shower, I use shampoo and conditioner from Garnier, although I don't wash it every day. I tame my hair with a Mason Pearson bristle brush. In the winter, I also use a Japanese wood comb to help cut down on winter static.

For cuts, a friend of mine, Carole Ramer, comes to the studio. We met through Angel Estrada, a designer who passed away from AIDS a while back. Carole used to work in a salon, but now she only does house calls. I used to have hair way past my waist and I did for many, many years. Then I wore it really short like Ruben's and then let it grow again. Five years ago, I settled on the length I have now. Carole is really incredible. She layers just the ends, and when she works, it's like she's cutting chiffon.

OTHER SERVICES

I don't go out for services. I do my own nails and prefer clear or sheer noncolors from OPI. Facials, I also do at home with those SK-II paper masks. They're fantastic; they help mellow my skin while I nap before a big night out. And I get a great foot massage from my husband!

DIET AND FITNESS

What you eat is what you look like. I don't eat fast food, and I cook at home. I'll cook a lot on the weekends, make soups and different kinds of beans, so I have food when I get home from work. As far as fitness, I hula hoop. I have since I was a kid, and it sort of puts me in a trance. I can hula for hours on my terrace. I do love a good bike ride through the countryside when time allows. I also highly recommend wearing a belt if you like a small waistline. It's great for maintaining a strong core, which helps with your posture. Otherwise, I walk a lot. I walk the several blocks to work and then up and down the stairs at the studio all day. Most important is to walk, walk, walk.

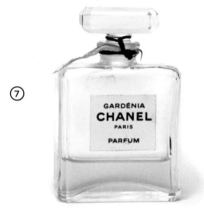

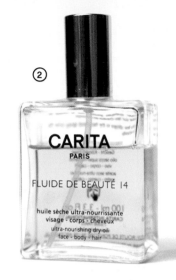

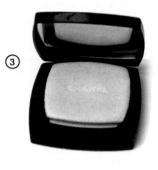

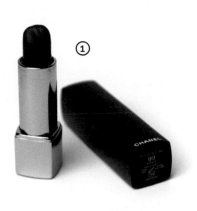

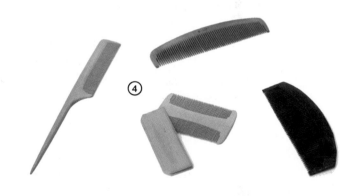

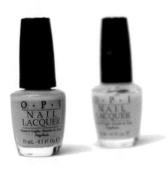

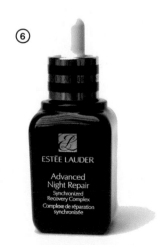

1 **Chanel**
Rouge Allure in
99 - Pirate

2 **Carita**
Fluide de Beauté 14

3 **Chanel**
compact

4 **Mason Pearson**
wood combs

5 **OPI** nail lacquer

6 **Estée Lauder**
Advanced Night
Repair

7 **Chanel** Gardénia

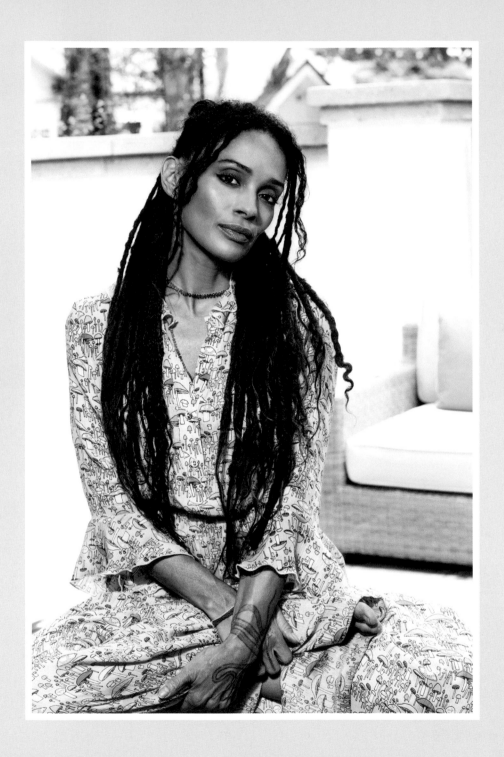

Lisa Bonet

Actress

SKIN CARE

A couple of times a week at least, I use pretty active things at night to keep the cells turning over. I use a scrub by my facialist Dayle Breault, or I'll use Derma Peel by Rhonda Allison. I'll alternate between the two. For cleansing, especially in the morning when I'm looking to sweep the dead cells away, I'll use Dayle's face soap or Rhonda Allison's Pumpkin Cleanser.

Then I'll use a couple of serums. I'll switch back and forth between Dayle's Truthful Serum or Le Mieux TGF-B Booster. I'll change it according to whatever my skin is needing that day. Then I'll use Dayle's spritz just to push the serums in deeper. I owe a lot to Dayle for my sustained youthfulness. I heard of her years ago through word of mouth. I've always taken skin care very seriously. From when I was a kid and would go to the drugstore and buy that Apricot Scrub, it was always important to me. I also have really sensitive skin that requires a good amount of care. I'm not one of those people who can go to sleep with their makeup on and wake up and be fine.

MAKEUP

I use a tinted sunblock by Epicuren, and I add a squirt of Sormé liquid concealer and mix that together. Zoë, my daughter, also has turned me onto this glow-y highlighter—it's Laura Mercier

Tinted Moisturizer Illuminating. I'll use Dr. Hauschka Tinted Day Cream on my eyes; it moisturizes lids and looks pretty. That's basically what I wear during the day. If I'm going out at night, I usually pick my eyes to accentuate. My go-to is a black sparkly pencil by Sisley. For me, it adds a little sparkle and it's very easy to play with. I'll use Shiseido mascara. And I have this very beautiful gold shadow by Dior. If I need it, I might use Clé de Peau concealer.

My brows are natural. I guess I got lucky. If you overtweeze, they might not grow back. I've always kept them quite full. Although, as young women we like to experiment—I did tweeze them once. I have one school picture for proof; it's amazing how brows can change your face. I remember my mother was flabbergasted when I came out of the bathroom. I would tell my daughters not to overtweeze—maybe Zoë did it once before—but you've got to let them fly too.

HAIR

I have had my hair in dreadlocks for a really long time. It's probably been twenty-something years now. I chose it and went for it because I really couldn't stand the amount of hours of tending and unraveling my hair. My hair would knot up pretty easily, and I don't like going to salons. It just seemed the natural solution. It's hilarious because people who don't know about dreads always wonder, "Do you wash your hair?" The answer is "Of course."

I usually use the Wen Cleansing Conditioner. If I'm looking for a really deep clean, then I'll use the Phyto products. After I wash, I'll also oil my hair up. If I don't add oil or if I overwash, my hair can become brittle. I like the Weleda Rosemary Conditioning Hair Oil, and I'll use organic coconut oil, which is also what I use on my body as well. I was using coconut oil before the current craze. It's simple and pure. Why put a lotion on your body that has ten ingredients when you can put on one that is from nature and smells divine and does the job?

FRAGRANCE

I usually stick with essential oils. There's a wonderful company called Living Libations and they have a fine, fine selection. They're based in Canada. I actually heard Nadine, one of the founders, speak at a breast health symposium, and I got turned onto her wealth of knowledge and was led to her company. I love her breast oil as well.

I might not tell you all the essential oils I use—you do have to keep a little mystery!—but you can't go wrong with rose and there's a beautiful gardenia too. I also like the neroli. I tend to gravitate toward more of the flower essential oils.

OTHER SERVICES

I'm a very, very big believer in bodywork. I have a few practitioners I see on a weekly basis. I'm relying on their skills, but these are bold, brave people who can go very deep. I've got quite a few different injuries over the years, and I use the bodywork to heal.

DIET AND FITNESS

I'm all about putting food in my body that nourishes me. I feel very lucky because so much is acceptable for diet here in L.A. There's the best of the best really. I used to be more skeptical about the gluten-free thing, but then one day, my daughter Lola had a cough, and she'd wake up in the middle of the night. It got worse and worse and the doctor had to give her an inhaler. Well, my own doctor had suggested that maybe it was gluten. We took the gluten away, and it's been such a big change. I pay for a gluten-free sourdough bread that gets baked fresh every week. A typical breakfast at home would be seasoned bone broth from Real Food Devotee, scrambled eggs cooked in coconut oil, and the sourdough bread toasted with raw butter.

My favorite form of fitness is dance. I take an African dance class here that I live for.

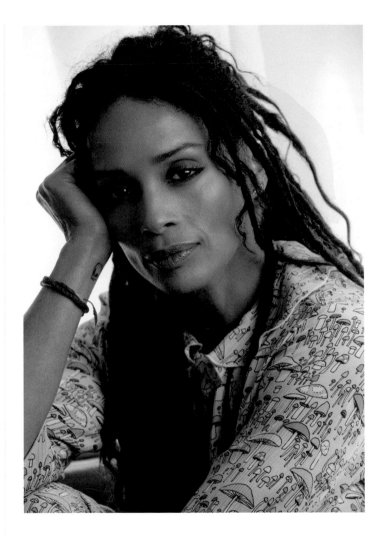

I just walked in one day and I have been doing it pretty regularly for seven years now. I also do Pilates twice a week, yoga once a week, and I go to the gym twice a week. I've always been a pretty physical person.

I was a gymnast when I was very young. I ran track and field and cross-country when I was in school. I probably would have been an athlete if I didn't become an artist.

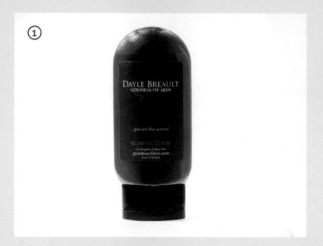

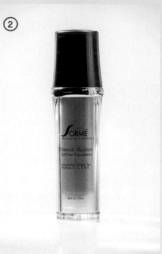

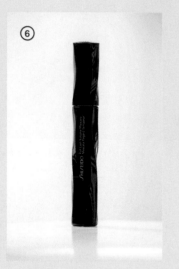

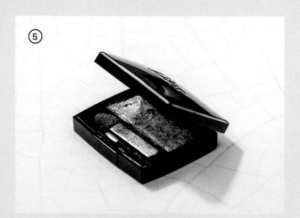

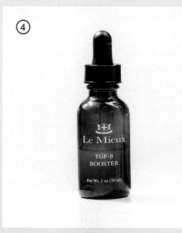

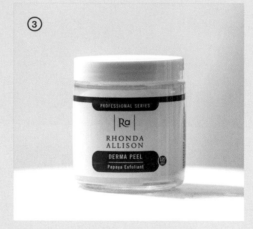

1 Dayle Breault
Bonifide Scrub

2 Sormé
Mineral Illusion
Oil-Free Foundation

3 Rhonda Allison
Derma Peel

4 Le Mieux
TGF-B Booster

5 Dior eye shadow

6 Shiseido
Full Lash Volume
Mascara

VIVE LA FRANCE!

Women have been obsessed with the idea of French beauty for generations. Less clear is what exactly defines the category. Surely, there's a certain sense of effortlessness (tousled hair) and restraint (a bare face and scarlet lips), but there's also the implacable sense of *je ne sais quoi*. The French beauty traditions—focus on skin care and pharmacy culture—likely have something to do with it. Great products also can't hurt. These French beauty finds are cult classics for a reason.

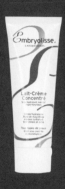
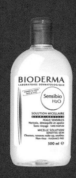
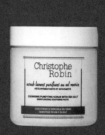
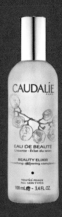

EMBRYOLISSE LAIT-CRÈME CONCENTRÉ

Before it became widely distributed, this rich cream was hoarded by makeup artists in Paris for fashion week. Cognac-born Laure Heriard Dubreuil, cofounder of the influential fashion retailer The Webster, always has it in her bag.

CHRISTOPHE ROBIN CLEANSING PURIFYING SCRUB WITH SEA SALT

Legendary colorist Christophe Robin originally created his mask to remove chemicals after a coloring session. Today, it's a terrific in-shower solution for boosting volume. Just ask Glossier founder Emily Weiss, who claims the sea salt gives her fine hair some texture.

BIODERMA SENSIBIO H2O

Perhaps the most popular product backstage at fashion weeks, this cleansing micellar water seems to magically remove stubborn makeup— even waterproof!—with a few doused cotton pads. Ellie Goulding is a fan.

CAUDALIE BEAUTY ELIXIR

This herbal-smelling mist is a regular on photo shoots. Particularly, a spritz or two revives midday makeup.

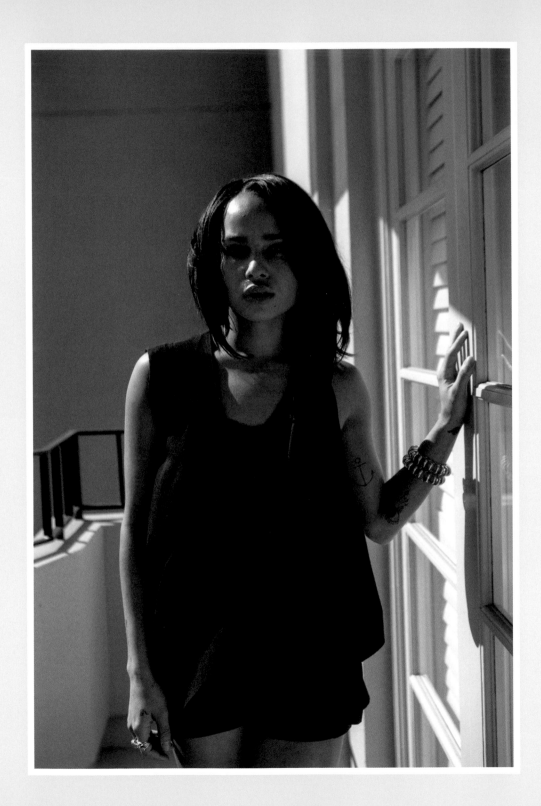

Zoë Kravitz

Actress and Musician

SKIN CARE

My morning and nighttime routines are pretty much the same. My facialist, Dayle Breault, who I've been going to since I was fifteen—my mom and dad go to her too, which is how I found out about her—makes her own line. She has an amazing face wash that I use, or when I'm traveling, she has these really great cleansing pads, which are like a toner and cleanser in one. Undereye, I use a cream by Dr. Hauschka. Kiehl's has an avocado eye cream that's good too. In the wintertime, I might use Dayle's mist afterward, because it keeps your skin moisturized, and I like her serum. I'll add that when it gets so dry here. Skin care–wise, Dayle has changed my life.

In the shower, I use Dr. Bronner's almond soap. Kiehl's has a really great soap too that I'll switch to sometimes. It's called Kiehl's Aromatic Blends: Vanilla & Cedarwood. Afterward, I'll use coconut oil. I'll use any brand as long as it's 100 percent, and it's something that I'll pick up at the health food store. For the most part, everything I use is either by Dayle or it's on the natural side. I don't like to put too much on if I don't know what it is; the product is going in your pores every day. Like with coconut oil, you can literally eat it. I also like this company called Simply Divine Botanicals. Their products are organic. They make really great body butters, and they have a face wash I like too. I've been using their How Now Brown Cacao butter. It smells like chocolate—yummy.

MAKEUP

Day to day, I don't wear a lot of makeup. Dayle makes an SPF that's really great, or Laura

Mercier has these shimmery tinted moisturizers with SPF. In the summertime, you can put a layer on and it's glow-y and pretty.

I do always wear blush, but it's like a stain. I've been wearing the Benefit liquid one—it's called Benetint—since high school. For a while, I was much more into shading, like contour or bronzer, and sometimes in the winter, I'll switch to that. My lip balm is by Dr. Hauschka. For mascara, I'm not picky about brand. I just don't like waterproof mascara because it doesn't come off.

If I'm going out at night, I'll do more. I do like a cat eye. Chanel makes this great liquid liner. That's my favorite thing. Sometimes, I'll do a classic red lip or a dark brown, but it's more work to keep it together as the color wanders. For that, NARS has good chubby pencils. I have them in Cruella, a warm red, and a color called Dragon Girl. I like to mix them together. When I first started performing with my band, Lolawolf, I would do more of a look. But it's me and two guys who

could care less if I was getting dressed up, so now I pretty much do the same as I would anyway. Depending on where my skin is at, I might wear a foundation. I don't like a lot of coverage. I'll dab on Radiant Creamy Concealer by NARS where I need it. And there's something called Lycogel that I discovered when I was shooting in South Africa. I went to a spa and tried it out and liked it. It's not heavy.

FRAGRANCE

I love oils. Right now, I like vanilla musk, which I picked up at Whole Foods. But I'll have others, and I usually mix different scents. Sometimes, I'll add a sandalwood. I'm also really into a Tom Ford cologne called Tobacco Vanille. It probably can be unisex—it works on both men and women. Also, recently this woman was wearing Tom Ford Tuscan Leather, which is more masculine, and it smelled incredible.

HAIR

Nikki Nelms comes to my house and cuts my hair. I met her at a *W* magazine shoot about two years ago. She's really adventurous and comes up with ideas for me for events and stuff like that. This is my natural hair color right now. I colored it a couple years ago and it was kind of blonde. It looked really cool, but my hair couldn't handle it.

Otherwise, I use Wen products to wash my hair. The shampoo is really a conditioner and shampoo in one. It's especially for African-American hair because it doesn't strip it of all the oils. My mom introduced me to it. I've always had her there for good beauty advice. We're both beauty fans. My friends are always laughing at her and me because we're like witches with our potions and bottles and things.

OTHER SERVICES

Where I really spoil myself is my facials with Dayle. She's between L.A. and New York, and I try to go as often as I can.

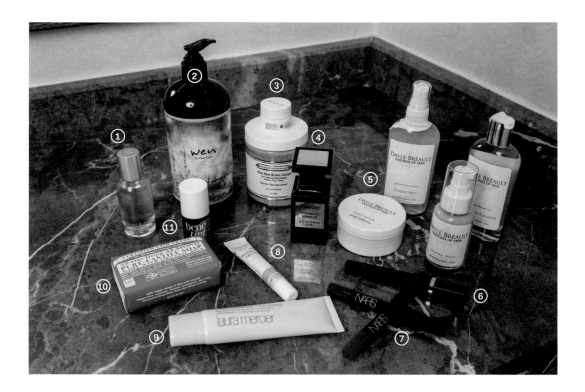

Her facials have also become my go-to gifts for girlfriends. My theory is when your skin is good, you can be confident and you don't have to wear makeup.

DIET AND FITNESS

I'm a big fan of juice and health and all that stuff. That's where beauty starts. I make sure that I'm eating well.

Usually for a film, I'll have to hit a gym. Although in the winter in New York, it can be tough to go out of the house. I go through phases. Right now, I really like the Ballet Beautiful at-home videos. I haven't been to an actual class of theirs in ages, but I'll travel with the videos, and you can do it anywhere. I do try to fit in cardio. In the summertime, I'll run in the park or something, and in the winter, it's the gym. I also walk everywhere. Thank god for New York, because I probably spend 80 percent of my time walking, from going up and down stairs to catching the subway.

1 **Kiehl's** Limited Edition Fragrance

2 **Wen** shampoo

3 **Simply Divine Botanicals** How Now Brown Cacao Butter

4 **Tom Ford** Tobacco Vanille Fragrance

5 **Dayle Breault** skin care products

6 Mascara

7 **NARS** Cruella and Dragon Girl lip pencils

8 **Dr. Hauschka** Daily Revitalizing Eye Cream

9 **Laura Mercier** Tinted Moisturizer

10 **Dr. Bronner's** Almond Soap

11 **Benefit** Benetint

ROSE-MARIE SWIFT
HOW TO CONTOUR AND HIGHLIGHT
LIKE A FASHION PRO

As with any trend that grabs hold and keeps hanging on, a look can start to look dated. For this generation, that trend may be contouring—shading with bronzer or a darker foundation in the hollows of the face, including under the cheekbones and down the sides of the nose. From contouring (or some might call it Kontouring, attributing the look to Kim Kardashian, who officially put it on the map) came its counterpoint: strobing, which is a fancy word for highlighting the elevated areas of the face like the tops of cheekbones and brow bones. But is there a way to incorporate both these ideas—they can be lovely and flattering when done well—and still look modern? For this challenge, I called on makeup artist Rose-Marie Swift, whose makeup M.O. might very well be fresh glow. She's known for a wonderful shimmering skin finisher from her own line, the beloved RMS Living Luminizer, and she has a cool, almost hippie approach to makeup that seems magically effortless.

Here's the thing about aggressive contouring and highlighting: It's not big anymore. If you look at all the campaigns and shows, people are going in a different direction. It's almost like a reality check. The drag queen makeup is not working. The truth is, no celebrity on the face of the earth wants to look like that. But why did it come about? Well, millennials wanted to connect to something that is theirs. And this contouring and highlighting, or strobing is what they call it, is happening all on social media. They are connecting with makeup stars on Instagram rather than your typical Elizabeth Arden or Estée Lauder. They're not interested in following the old school lessons.

But what they've done is process this all through an app that makes everything look flawless. That is not reality. When you walk down the street, that is not what you want to see. It's scary. When I see that, I think, "If someone hits you on the back of your head, your face will fall off."

That's not to say contour and highlighting can't be done in a beautiful way.

TIPS FOR FLATTERING DEFINITION AND HIGHLIGHTING

Start with Great Skin.

The look today, especially with the HD cameras, is all about healthy skin. This is why celebrities are all into their green juices and infrared saunas. This is really where you should start if you want succulent skin and that glow. No amount of highlighter can compensate for that.

Pick the Right Base.

That said, when it comes to your base, avoid clays and talc. They are thickening and building agents, and it would be like adding a layer of dirt over your lawn. Instead, look for sheer formulas. You can always build.

Contour.

I use creams. It looks more real on the skin, whereas powders can look dirty and flat. Put it under your cheekbone and aim the swipe to your nostrils. Some of these kids are drawing the contour down to the lips. I don't do that because it draws the face down and ages you.

Highlight.

The traditional way is to highlight the elevated areas of your face, such as the cheekbone, down the nose, bow of the lip, brow bone, and center of the eyelid. You can also highlight and skip the contour. One beautiful way to wear it is to wear only the highlighter, and you can get away with not wearing a lot of makeup. Ideally, you should pick a formula that you can still see your skin through. Color is also important when highlighting. If you're a black or brown girl, you don't want a whitish hue. Go for a rose gold or gold. For girls who are really pale, you can go in either direction, but it depends on what you're wearing.

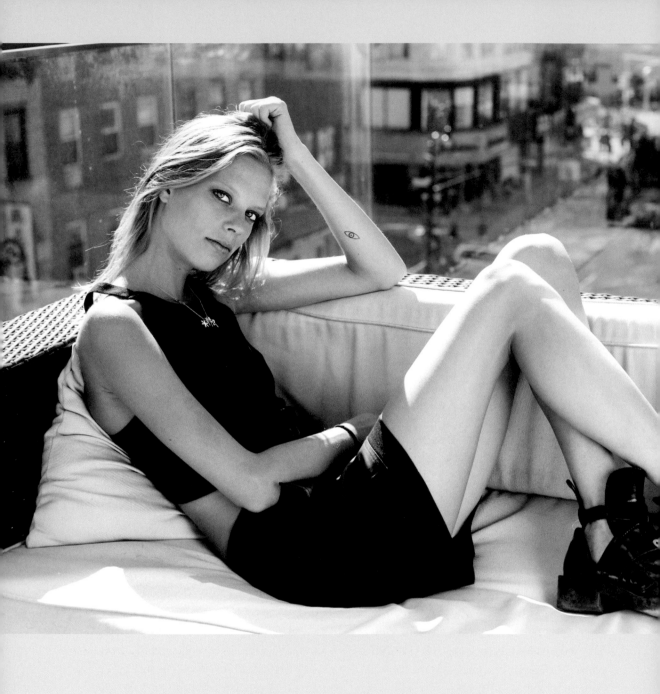

Lexi Boling

Model

SKIN CARE

I just use water to wash my face. I used to use all kinds of face washes, but then I would wind up irritated. I used water for three months and my skin cleared up and calmed down. And it's easy when you're traveling and stuff. Then I use Nerium day cream and also the eye serum—it wakes me up. I always wear sunscreen. I'm wearing SPF 50 right now, but if I'm not going to be outside a lot, I wear one from Neutrogena that has SPF 25.

At the end of the day, if I need it, I use the Chanel or Dior makeup remover. They each come in a big blue bottle and they're oil-based. It's great especially if I had to wear a smoky eye for a shoot or something like that. Then I use water to wash my face and the Age-Defying Night Cream from Nerium. I heard about the brand from my mom. She loves it and she has great skin.

If I get a breakout, I'll put some tea tree oil on it. It dries it out really well. My boyfriend taught me, funny enough.

MAKEUP

Where I grew up, it was about tanning beds, loads of makeup, and big hair. The look is definitely like a leather bag. Everybody is really tan all the time. My hair is super stringy and my mom would never let me go tanning. I was not the norm at all. But now, of course, I'm glad. My mom also would always say, "Less is more." When I'm not working, I try to keep my skin clear.

If I'm going out, then I'll put on a bit of Chanel foundation. I use a mascara from Gucci. I like it because the brush is not super hairy. Most people are about things like blush or lipstick, but contour/highlight is where it's at. I picked up highlighting from Pat McGrath and her team. When I first started doing runway, I would pay attention backstage to what she would do. She always uses a highlight, which makes everything look dewy. You need to look fresh. Now I use the rose-gold highlighter from her line. I put it above my cheekbone and on my temples. Then I'll use the Harry Brant for MAC contour palette. I met him through friends like Cat McNeil, another model.

FRAGRANCE

There's a lot to choose from in the Prada Candy line. I like the new one, Kiss. It's sort of sweet, but there's some musk to it. When shooting the campaign with Steven Meisel, it's wonderful because he sets this very relaxing atmosphere. When you get on set, he puts you in a chair and says, "Do you." Shooting beauty is different than fashion. Beauty, you try to show yourself through your eyes or face. You have to relax your features. Fashion it's more about your body, and you can go a bit more crazy. If you grew up in a small town like I did, where beauty was only one thing, it's cool to be working in beauty from a fashion standpoint. In fashion, you can be weird or edgy or cool and still be considered beautiful.

HAIR

My hair gets destroyed from all the styling. And last year, I dyed my hair black for one week and then had to go back to blonde. I had to get it bleached six times. I'm done coloring my hair; it's a natural dirty blonde now. I'm using Olaplex—the No. 3 one. Shampoo and conditioner, I use Redken. I also use the Redken Anti-Snap cream after the shower. Before fashion week and during, when I can, I'll use a bunch of masks. I like the Moroccanoil one that comes in a tub.

OTHER SERVICES

I just got hip surgery last month. I tore my labrum snowboarding. So right now, it's a lot of physical therapy. Hopefully it won't affect my walk. I'm doing therapy, and then I'm going to practice in heels. I'm hoping I can suffer through if it hurts.

DIET AND FITNESS

Diet is not really anything I think about. I'm six foot one. It's always been quite easy to stay thin. I eat chicken nuggets. I pretty much eat whatever I want. But if I'm feeling crappy, I'll go to hot yoga. The Victoria's Secret girls work out every single day. I don't know how they do it. But a lot of the times for the runway girls, they don't want us to work out because we can get too thin. I've been told that before actually. It's just finding a balance that works.

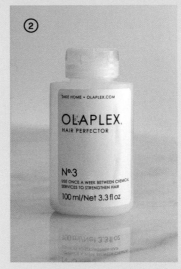

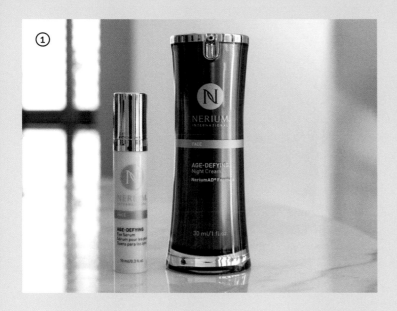

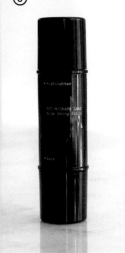

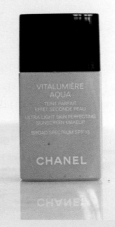

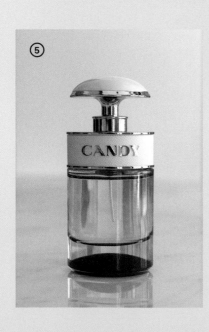

1 **Nerium**
Age-Defying Eye
Serum, Night Cream

2 **Olaplex**
No. 3 shampoo

3 **Pat McGrath Labs**
Nude Shiny Stick
Highlighter

4 **Chanel**
Vitalumiere Aqua
foundation

5 **Prada** Candy

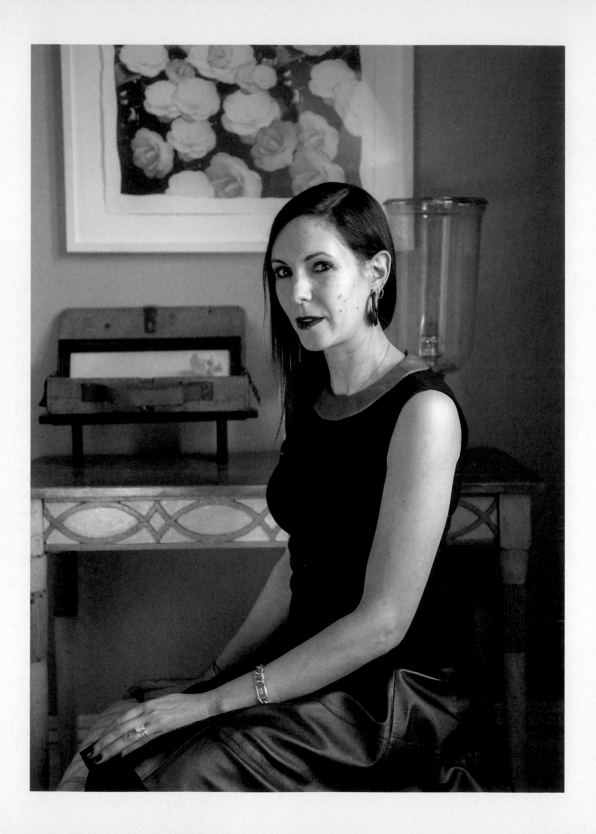

Jill Kargman

Author and Actress

SKIN CARE

Typically, I'll go to SoulCycle at 6 A.M., shower, and then start my day. For soap, I use Jo Malone Red Roses shower gel. I love it. You smell like Mena Suvari in that bathtub. For body lotion, I use Naked Body Butter from Bliss, which I steal from my husband. He's metrosexual.

Then, every day, I do this lotion called P50 1970 by Biologique Recherche. It's ridiculous sounding—you'd think it was a military nuclear bomb formula—and it smells beyond, like something you'd pour in your car engine. My husband actually hates it because of the smell, but I started using it a year ago and I haven't had a blackhead since. A friend of mine who has gorgeous skin was the one to tell me about it. I ran into her and was like, "Why do you look like a fetus?" She explained and I ran to get it. Now I don't use cleanser, just this.

Then I'll use a Shiseido brightening cream. I'm starting to get age spots. On top of that, I'll use Chanel Sublimage face cream. I used to do nothing and people used to call me Snow White. I loved that. That was about ten years ago; now nobody calls me that. I think it coincided with

having my third kid. Anyway, I started taking better care of myself.

I believe in the valor of pallor. I want to be even whiter. I've come to the conclusion that the only sunblock that works is a building. I used to wear sunblock every day, but after having melanoma, my doctor said you shouldn't even be in the sun at all. Now on the beach, I'm shrouded like a ninja. When I ski, I wear a ski mask. In the city, I walk on the shady side of the street. I should be a P.I. because I skulk in the shadows.

Before I go to bed, I'll use the P50 again and redo the creams. Also, a couple times a week, I do a Shiseido brightening mask or one from SK-II. They're those paper masks, and when you put it on you look like a serial killer. I've terrified my kids a few times.

MAKEUP

During the day, I don't wear that much. I'll use concealer if I have eye bags, and I've been getting MAC Face and Body Foundation in white. I'll use it to smooth everything out. It's not available in department stores, only at MAC's professional store. They're often sold out, and sometimes when I schlep all the way there, they take pity on me and give me a big sample. Then I'll use NARS Crystal Setting Powder. It helps me attain my Kabuki status. For lips, I'll use lip gloss or a sheer lip tint from Flower, which is Drew Barrymore's line. Sometimes, I'll do Chanel instead in Summer Plum, which is also a gloss. My lips are too dry to wear lipstick ever.

I never wear blush. I don't want any color on my skin. I want to look like a dead body. My beauty icon is Madame X. I also skip the mascara because I get falsies. I do wear this NARS eye pencil, which is black with sparkles in it. I'll only put it on the water line because I have both bottom and top eyeliner tattooed on. I love my eyeliner tattoos because I'll be at the gym at 5:30 in the morning and it looks like I just woke up like this.

In the evening, I might put on a heavier application of the MAC Face and Body white, and Flower has the best stuff called Color Play Cream eyeshadow and you just shove your finger in the pot. I like dark colors like charcoal or midnight or black glitter.

FRAGRANCE

I have the Jo Malone Red Roses cologne, and I have the Bulgari perfume, the yellow one.

HAIR

I'm practically bald. I used to have such good hair, but it was like a Jewfro. But then with each child, it got successively worse. It was like a nightmare in a shower drain. That's why I started taking biotin in megadoses—we're talking handfuls. I also go to Philip Kingsley for treatment. It's usually bald Wall Street guys who want their hair back and Jill. I also use his shampoo, the green one for itchy scalps. It's great.

For the last eight years, I've been getting my hair cut by Stefanie at Frédéric Fekkai in The Mark, which I love, because it's like a secret hideaway. Jessica there colors my hair black with a blue tint in it. I want to look like Veronica of "Betty and Veronica." I used to have really long hair, but I had a midlife crisis at thirty-five and chopped eight inches off my hair and got two tattoos. For me, I feel younger with short hair. Now, to quote Stefanie, it's "collar-bone dusting."

OTHER SERVICES

I go to Aida Bicaj for my facials. I don't go regularly because I'm house-broke from my move; we're moving to a place just a few blocks away. I probably go about three times a year. There's also this Chinese massage place down the street that I'm obsessed with. It's only $55 for the hour, and they have more talent than any of these $250 spa places. They beat you down. You hear the other people moaning and you think it's a happy ending, but it's not. They're also so nice.

For nails, I'll have my manicure at Fekkai while I'm having my hair done. I only do Shellac. With three kids, their activities, and bath time, I could never keep a color on before. Now, I love my nails blood red. My nails haven't seen sunlight in three years.

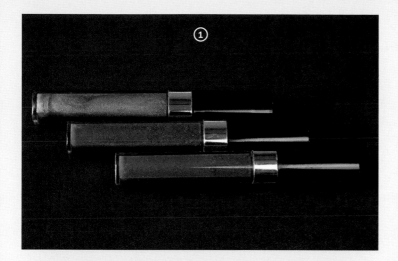

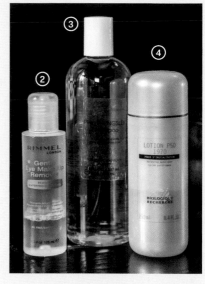

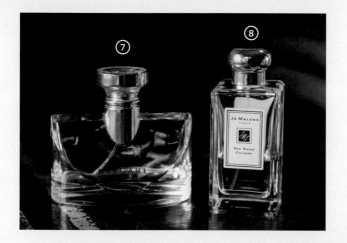

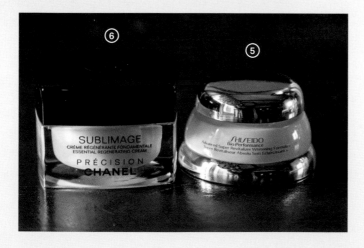

1 **Chanel**
lip glosses

2 **Rimmel** Gentle Eye
Makeup Remover

3 **Philip Kingsley**
shampoo

4 **Biologique
Recherche**
Lotion P50 1970

5 **Shiseido**
Bio-Performance

6 **Chanel**
Sublimage

7 **Bulgari**
fragrance

8 **Jo Malone**
Red Roses Cologne

PATRICIA WEXLER
ON BOTOX and AGING

When it comes to aging, female celebrities have it rough. Let things happen completely naturally and you might age yourself out of roles. But overdo the interventions and you become a cautionary tale to younger actresses. The damned if you do, damned if you don't dichotomy is where dermatologists like Patricia Wexler, M.D., come in. I love hearing her stories, which are some of the best in the business—all without naming names of course. She's been around long enough to have seen the mistakes cosmetic dermatology has made and how far methods have come. Particularly, Botox is an area that was once white hot—hence, often overused—but is now receiving some celebrity backlash. But Patricia thinks the neurotoxin still has a place in anti-aging regimens.

I never thought I would be a dermatologist with celebrity clients. I was actually an infectious disease consultant. I was one of the first people to work on HIV. All of my patients were dying, and then, at the same time, my parents were both dying. I couldn't deal with everything being so negative, so I went back to training. I went back to dermatology and finished in 1986. There was no cosmetic dermatology then except for dermabrasion.

I opened my first office in a basement in the Village in '86. One of my first patients was Paulina Porizkova. It was a week before she did *Sports Illustrated*, and she had a rash. We resolved that, and she started referring other models and actresses and it just went from there. I never had press in the beginning; it was just word of mouth. I was interested in the new things coming out. I was one of the first people in New York to do Botox cosmetically. I did liposuction in '86 before it was popular.

The field has changed, of course. Before cosmetic dermatology, people went straight to surgery. When I started, women would come and say, I don't want to look like so and so. It was because the work she had done was so obvious. And the problem with bad surgery is that it ages badly. Good surgery you don't even notice. My philosophy became to start addressing skin early so a lot of people will never need to have surgery.

Here's how I approach aging: If you're sixty and want to look thirty, that's not happening. You'll just look like you're trying to be thirty. It's far better to be sixty and look wonderful at that age because you're taking care of yourself. It's about aging gracefully by doing the little things all the time.

Don't Start Botox Too Young

People are easily living into their eighties now. If you start Botox in your twenties, your facial muscles are going to get thin. If you do it the forehead and that muscle thins, then the skin overlying the muscle is going to get looser. So to do it before you see wrinkles doesn't make any sense. I believe in starting when you start seeing wrinkles in rest.

Don't Freeze Your Face

I have some actresses who do nothing when they're working because they want to look natural and have expressions on screen. In their private life, though, they might do a tiny bit of Botox or filler here and there. You don't want to be expressionless. You want a certain amount of movement because people relate to emotion. The joke around the office is that you don't want all these children traumatized by their nonsmiling mothers.

Don't Use Botox for the Wrong Reasons

People often use Botox for the wrong reasons. For example, you get crow's feet because you lose volume in the area. You need to replace the volume first and see how it comes out. If you use too much Botox in the cheek, your cheek is going to abruptly stop. It's called the Botox shelf. That's when you see these women with the little apples on their cheeks. Or if you're using the neurotoxin in the lines between the eyes, called the "11s," you're going to get a lift of the brow. You have to make sure it suits your face—and you're not just looking constantly surprised.

Be Open to Multiple Appointments

If I do the "11s," I'll first put in a tiny bit of neurotoxin and then bring the patient back ten days later. That way you can leave the maximum amount of movement while still looking great. The idea is not to freeze somebody but to reduce overexpression from lines.

Leave Yourself Room for Mistakes

If you have a big event, you'll want to schedule your appointment two weeks earlier. The neurotoxin will peak at one week. You want it to relax a little before the event. You also want that buffer because you might bruise. It's always a possibility even if you never bruised before.

Unexpected Ways of Using Botox

I've treated some women with Botox in the underarm—it prevents sweating there. It's usually for a wedding or the red carpet. You see how hot it is in L.A. all the time? There's nothing worse than sweating through when you're wearing a silk gown. If you do Botox under the arm, you get about six months of no perspiration there. For men, we might do it on the forehead, not because of wrinkles but because they don't want to be mopping their head on the red carpet from sweat.

Another thing is women are getting Botox on their hairline. They call it 'Blow-tox.' Because it stops you from perspiring there, you can preserve your blow outs longer because you don't have to wash as much.

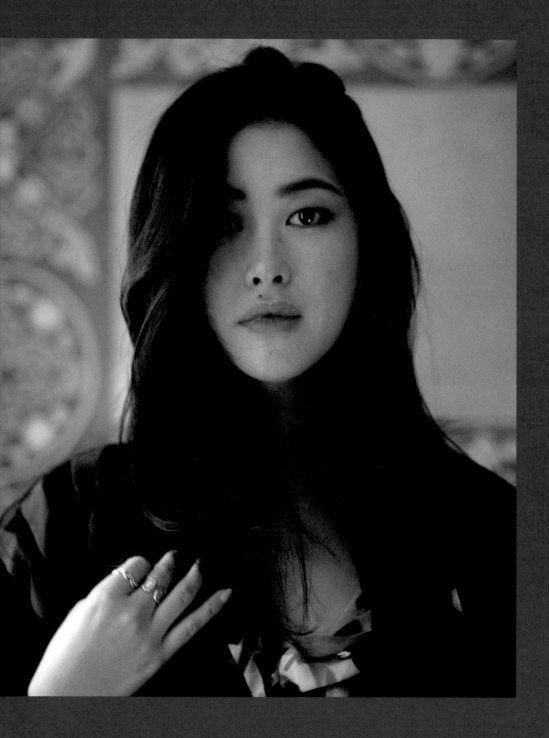

Zhu Zhu

Actress

SKIN CARE

I wake up and go brush my teeth. Lately, I've been using this toothpaste I quite like called Splat Professional. I feel like its good for my teeth and gums. I don't know even know where it's from, maybe Russia. The paste itself is actually kind of burgundy.

Then, I use Shu Uemura cleansing oil to wash my face, which is great because my skin is dry. Probably twice or three times a week, I'll exfoliate. I like the exfoliator by Clarins—it's very,

very light, so you could even use it every day if you wanted. And lately, I found another product made from white rice that's by Origins. That's pretty good too. After, I'll use the Chanel Hydra Beauty Essence Mist. I'll use it before I put on my skin care products and sometimes to finish and set my makeup. It makes your skin look really dewy—it's a favorite.

Then, a lot of girls here would use serums. But I don't want to burden my face with too much product. I'll save the serums for when I'm older. Right now, I'm in love with Crème de la

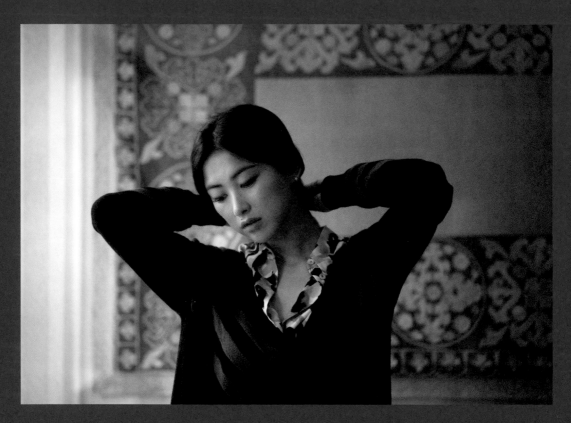

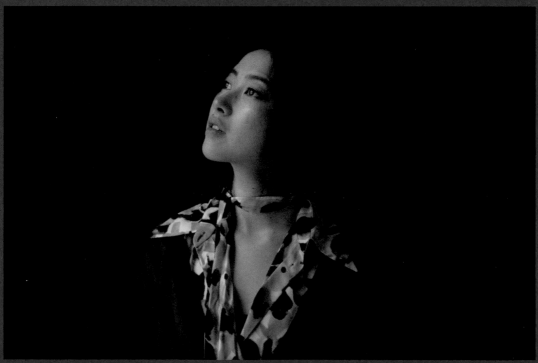

Mer. When my skin is in good condition, I'll put on just a light application. I pat it in. Sunblock is by Clarins—it's the little white bottle that you have to shake. I don't use any eye cream. I just use whatever I put on my face under my eyes.

At night, the routine is similar. Sometimes I'll do a mask if I feel like I had a lot of makeup on that day or was out in the sun. I like a hydrogen mask—it's an easy one and it's supposed to soothe and relax your skin. It also feels a little bit cold on, which is nice. You can pick it up at any of the local pharmacies here, and any Korean or Japanese brand works. There's a lot of skin care out of Korea and definitely Korean women care about their skin. But I'm not one of those Asian girls that go crazy about skin care. I just do a simple routine.

MAKEUP

My makeup choices are from years of shopping and experience. I've bought many wrong products. I've paid for my "lessons." Now I've settled on what works for me. I like the MAC Face and Body Foundation. Sometimes, it can't even cover all my flaws, but I like it because it looks really natural and it evens out my skin tone. I try to keep my application light. Beijing is very dry so I don't like to use too much foundation. The product can dry up and flake, and also my skin is very dry so I can't carry a lot of makeup.

And then I do a little taupe eye shadow. I'm not really specific on brands but I like NARS eye shadows. I also like shimmery ones by Dior, but that's more for evening. I curl my lashes and put on mascara. Then I put on a little bit of blush, which is by Bobbi Brown—the Shimmer Brick compact in Rose. The color is super light, but it just brightens up your face. And then some lip balm: Eight Hour Cream by Elizabeth Arden.

At night, I'll probably add black eyeliner. I like the ones by Japanese brands like Kanebo or Shiseido. They're very soft and very thin, so the line is almost delicate after you apply it. Maybe for eye shadows I'll go a few shades darker for a smoky eye. Or if I do a simple eye, I'll do straight, thicker eyebrows and a red lip. My eyebrows are naturally pretty thick. I like to brush them with this gel by Bobbi Brown that looks like mascara. Then I'll use a little bit of liquid brow pen by Japanese brand Kate. The color almost comes off like a tattoo.

FRAGRANCE

I love Jo Malone. I got the Orange Blossom scent as a gift from a friend of mine many years ago, and I fell in love with it. It's very light, natural, sweet—it's there but not that obvious.

HAIR

For shampoo and conditioner, I also use Jo Malone. I use the Lime Basil & Mandarin scent. It's really spa-ish.

I have really long hair, so I don't cut it all that often. Sometimes, when I'm working, I just have the stylist on set trim it for me. I don't have a salon I go to. I also don't dye my hair. When I was a teenager, I dyed my hair five colors at one time. It was all different shades of red going from more orange to more purple. But I was young and bold then. I thought I looked so cool! But I would never do it again.

SERVICES

Nails, I haven't done colors or gels for a long time because of *Marco Polo*, because it's set in ancient Mongolia—they probably didn't have nail polish! Before that, I would sometimes get gels because the color stays longer. I like the French manicure style, or I'll go with nude or red.

For massages, I go to Chinese medicine doctors and they do deep tissue and medical massages. It has the best results. I've been to Swiss or French spas, and the massages are really nice and comforting and soothing and all that, but I feel like after my Chinese medicine massages my body functions better. It helps with circulation.

Facials, I don't go very often, because if you go too often it makes your skin sensitive. There's a small Korean spa in Beijing that I go to. I just follow a specific woman named Ping and I see her there.

DIET AND FITNESS

I do pay attention to both diet and fitness, but I eat whatever I want. Sometimes, I think, "I've got to quit carbs," or something like that, but I never do. I think life is difficult enough; you have to treat yourself well. I do try to control the amount of what I eat—no huge portions. And I try to chew more and chew slowly. Each bite, I chew maybe thirty-five to forty times. That works.

I don't really go to gyms, but I swim, I run outside in parks, and I ride horses. I ride at my uncle's stable, which is a horse-riding club. I actually learned how to ride when I was six, but I stopped for many years. But then with shooting *Marco Polo*—we were doing the battle scenes in Kazakhstan and it's the most amazing landscape ever—I fell in love with it all over again.

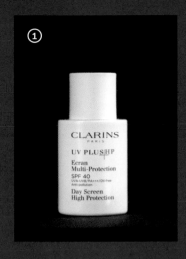

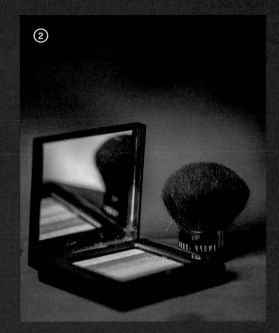

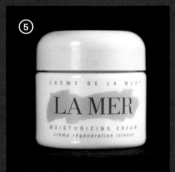

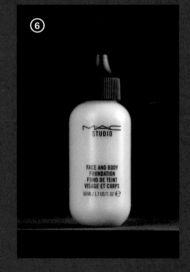

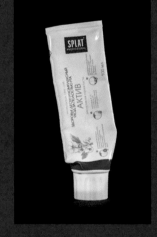

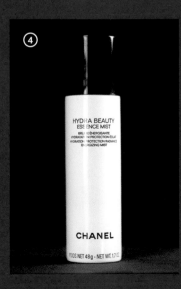

1	**Clarins** sunblock	4	**Chanel** Hydra Beauty Essence Mist
2	**Bobbi Brown** Shimmer Brick Compact in Rose	5	**La Mer** Crème de la Mer
3	**Splat Professional** Toothpaste	6	**MAC** Face and Body Foundation

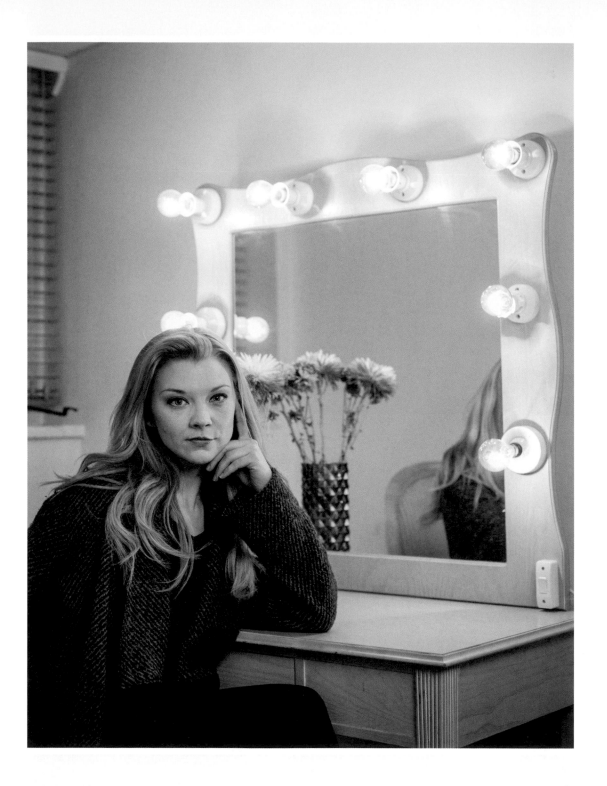

Natalie Dormer

Actress

SKIN CARE

If I'm shooting that morning, the first things that go on my face (especially the case if I'd been to an event the night before and had one too many glasses of champagne!) are these Hydro Cool Firming Eye Gels by Skyn Iceland. It helps tame the puffiness. Then I'll down a glass of tepid lemon water—I've been doing that since I was a student.

At the moment, I love the Ole Henriksen Truth Serum Collagen Booster. It's got a vitamin C complex in it, and I've been putting that on every morning and night for the last couple of months.

For body moisturizer, I use whatever I've been given—I've been gifted a lot of body lotion, and I spend so much time in hotels. I'm a Brit, so there will always be some Molton Brown and the Body Shop products in there. I also like this great body oil by Ila that I'll put under my moisturizer if my skin is very dry. The oil permeates. I saw that when I was filming *Game of Thrones* in Morocco. The women of that country love their argan oil, and I picked up the idea of putting on an oil or oily serum before moisturizer.

At night, I do more. If I'm coming off set— right now I'm shooting *Patient Zero*, and we're running around with this face gel makeup on, and there's no ventilation at all—the best way to take off all that pretend makeup is the Elemis Pro-Collagen Cleansing Balm. I rub it all over my face and then use a hot flannel and wipe off the day's makeup. I'll do the Henriksen serum and then I've been using the Cowshed Quinoa moisturizer. And for years, I have loved the Dermalogica Multivitamin Recovery Masque. It's amazing if your skin is extra tired or you've been on one too many long-haul flights. Or like when I was training for the London Marathon—I ran it last year—I was doing some of my running when I was in New York. The wind coming off the Hudson River is incredible! Your face takes a battering. This is super hydrating for situations like that. And good old-fashioned Vaseline is great for lips, and I'll put a little under the bra straps if I'm doing long runs to stop the friction.

MAKEUP

La Prairie Skin Caviar is my foundation. I adore it. It was put on me a decade ago, and I have never strayed from it. It's got an SPF 15 in it, but if I'm somewhere hot or with bright sun I'll put on a stronger SPF around my eye area, on my cheekbones, and the end of my nose. Natura Bisse makes a good one called Diamond White with an SPF 50. The Make Up For Ever concealer is also magic. I always have one in my bag.

When it comes to my eyebrows, I'm a MAC girl. I use the pencil, and I've also been using the MAC Fluidline liner for years. I have very particularly shaped almond-y eyes, so I have trouble finding mascara that doesn't drop on me. The Clinique High Impact mascara doesn't bleed.

For the rest, I'm a little bit of a flirt because I get put in makeup so much. Maybe I'll be working with a makeup artist that has a great relationship with NARS or Lancôme and then I'll use those things. I just got some beautiful eyeshadow palettes from Lancôme. They are all color coordinated so it's easy. When I'm not working, I'm not really a lip girl. I might go for a stain, but that's about it.

FRAGRANCE

My signature scent is the old Gucci by Gucci before they reimagined it. I was really upset when they discontinued it, but there's a funny story. My sister's boyfriend is in the navy, and he managed to find like six bottles on the U.S. base in Bahrain. He sent me a text and I told him to buy all of them! He's a British naval officer and there he is at the U.S. station buying up all the Gucci bottles. I've got maybe two years' worth of it now!

HAIR

I had to shave a side of my hair for *The Hunger Games*, and I'm trying to grow it out. I'm taking Solgar Wild Alaskan omega capsules so it'll grow in strong. I think it's working—I've got a couple inches growing on my undercut. I'm not picky about shampoo, but I love the Fekkai hair mask. I also like to put a little bit of Moroccanoil in my hair occasionally. My hair color is actually completely natural—a dirty blonde. I've got Norwegian blood.

SERVICES

I have an amazing masseuse—I don't want to give away her name; she's very private. I see her probably once a week; she lives really close to me and I just go over to her. As an actor, it's weird because you end up with all these different strains. Maybe

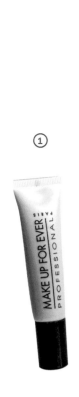

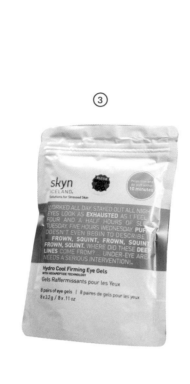

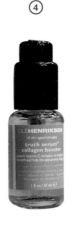

1 **Make Up For Ever**
Concealer

2 **Clinique** High
Impact Mascara

3 **Skyn Iceland**
Hydro Cool
Firming Eye Gels

4 **Ole Henriksen**
Truth Serum
Collagen Booster

I've been squeezed to death in a corset, or when I was doing *Mockingjay 2* I was carrying a big semiautomatic rifle over my shoulder and it made me really lopsided. Going to her also helps when my running injuries kick in. When I can, I really like going to the Corinthia spa in London.

I also treat myself at home. It's important to get a foam roller and really limber yourself up. I also love Tiger Balm and Epsom salts for when I'm running, or just all your aches and pains.

DIET AND FITNESS

In Britain, they teach a yoga lesson every day when you're in drama school. It's mandatory if you're doing classical training. The idea is that you're trying to break things down physically as well as emotionally and to get rid of all those habits and tensions in your body. That's my primary source of exercise now. There will always be a yoga mat in my luggage, period. Running is my second source. For me, it's more of a mental exercise.

It's also a really good way of discovering a new city. I'm hoping to run the New York City Marathon in November.

I'm pretty balanced in what I eat. I also drink a ton of water. The old rules are the best rules. Every woman knows that. And I love to sleep. I can catch an extra twenty minutes anywhere. I always say Dormer, *dormir*, it's very similar.

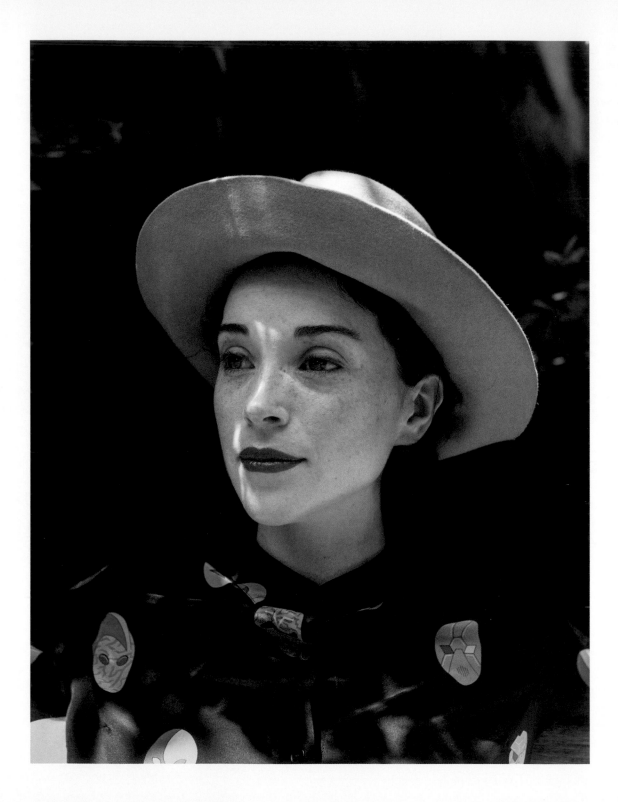

St. Vincent

Musician

SKIN CARE

I wash my face with a Dayle Breault wash—she's a facialist that a friend of mine recommended and she lives just a block away in the East Village. And then I put on SPF. I always wear SPF; I'm very fair, so I freckle and burn. I've been vacillating between a Neutrogena one from SuperTarget and Kiehl's. That's it. I'm very, very low maintenance, bordering on extreme laziness.

In the shower, I use Dr. Bronner's. I like the lavender scent, but I'm usually in hotels, so I just use whatever shower gels and whatever body lotions are available.

If I just played a show, I have some sort of Kiehl's eye makeup remover, and then I use the same face wash. For moisturizer, I use the Egyptian Magic stuff. It's not too heavy for me.

MAKEUP

If it's just day-to-day, I try to get away with wearing as little as possible. I have a Laura Mercier Tinted Moisturizer that I'll use on my face. And

I've been using the pink-and-green Maybelline mascara that I get from SuperTarget—I love it there, I go whenever I'm in Dallas—since I was thirteen. I also have a red lipstick from a drugstore in Paris that has served me well. It's by a brand called Mavala.

Of course, for events and performances, it's fun to play around. We do our own makeup on tour. I try to pick up tips whenever I can. Such as, go about 10 percent more when you're going onstage than you would in your day-to-day. I also tend to wear a lot of black onstage, so it's good to have a little bit of color. I do still stick to my Laura Mercier Tinted Moisturizer. I'm not wearing heavy foundation onstage, ever, even though maybe I should. For a while, I was doing a Laura Mercier blue shadow. I just went to MAC, though, and got some really bold matte colors that I'm going to try. I like textures. Although any dewiness you see is probably just a product of sweating—I guarantee you that's not intentional. My eyebrows, sometimes I fill them in with this crayon my bandmate gave me. I've bleached them before when I was blonde. It made me look like a very nice person. There's something really sweet about a light brow.

I'm really excited for Governors Ball. I worked with Phoebe English on some custom looks for the show. I'll be coordinating the beauty to those looks, but it's more instinct and going in the moment than completely planned out. I have gotten more interested in experimenting lately. Sometimes it's a failure, sometimes it's a hit. It's a funny nexus of obviously a certain amount of vanity because you're acknowledging you're going on stage and asking people to look at you, but then you can just have fun with it. It's makeup; it's not going to cure cancer.

HAIR

Growing up in Dallas, sure, there are beauty stereotypes, but I didn't have the chance to fit into any of them. It's mostly all about being tan and having straight blonde hair. I didn't really have an "in" in that regard. But I didn't worry about it too much. It's a very specific Texas style, but it's not unilateral. My hair is naturally very curly and dark; it's been through a lot. Earlier in the year, I had silvery lavender hair. There wasn't a specific reference. Pamela Neal out in Los Angeles, who did David Bowie and does Björk's hair and basically everyone in the world who I think is cool, did it. I came in with a mess of hair and she took a look and brought out this lavender wash. It was spontaneous. It was definitely a punk rock–guerilla style moment. Flying by the seat of my pants and being in the moment, that's what makes beauty fun.

Pamela is responsible for the highlighted mullet I had at Coachella too. I got an unfortunate *Grease* haircut in Dallas over the holidays that I like to call "Audrey Hepburn with an anger problem." Pamela did the best she could do with it. Then I had really unfortunate boy-band frosted tips—it was a *look*. But I think it's fun when things look kind of silly.

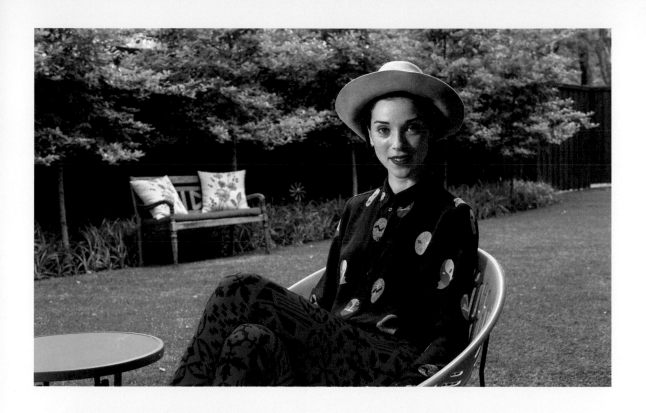
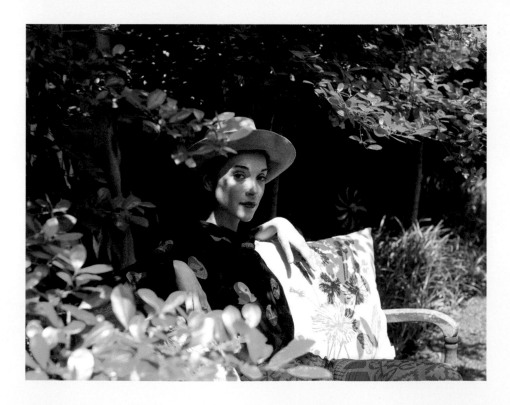

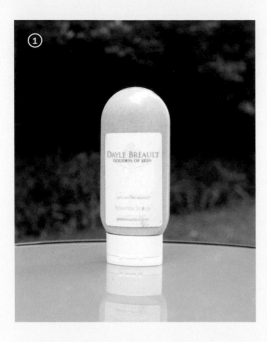

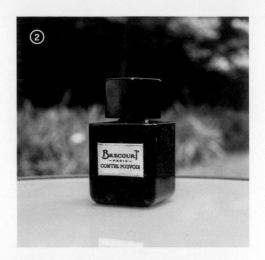

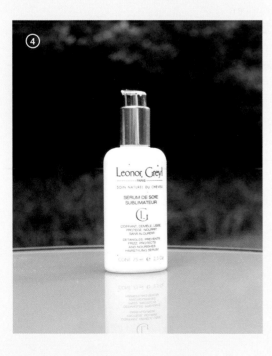

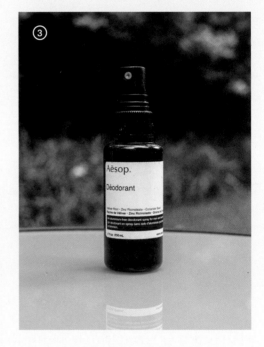

1 **Dayle Breault**
face wash

2 **Brecourt**
Contre Pouvoir
fragrance

3 **Aesop**
Deodorant

4 **Leonor Greyl**
Serum de Soie

Now, I don't really know what it is. I have long fringe that starts at the crown of my head but then it's really curly in the back. For events, I've been straightening it and slicking it back. It's also back to dark, and there's about two-and-a-half inches of actually natural color that's healthy and still about two inches of the boy-band frosted tips that's been dyed over. I'm just going to go into the salon and say I want the "Nick Cave" minus the receding hairline.

With all this, my hair is pretty fry guy. I've been using a Leonor Greyl mask. It comes in a square bottle, it's really heavy, and it takes up a lot of space in the suitcase. There should be beluga caviar in it for what it takes to lug around. But it's the only thing that's been helping me grow my hair out.

FRAGRANCE

I got a tincture of some lavender-y thing from a friend who's really into essential oils. And I like the Aesop deodor-ant; I like to use it as perfume. I also got a man-scent when I was in Amsterdam called Brecourt Contre Pouvoir that I like.

OTHER SERVICES

I get massages on tour a lot because the show is very active and holding a guitar for two hours a day has done a number on my back alignment.

DIET AND FITNESS

I do run and lift weights and, of course, I have the show. I've always been very active. I grew up doing sports, and I don't like to sit down. I'm usually at hotels, so I just run at the gyms there. But I actually never exercise if I'm in NYC. Then I just ride a bike around, but that's not really exercise. It's not very strenuous.

Diet? Pass on that.

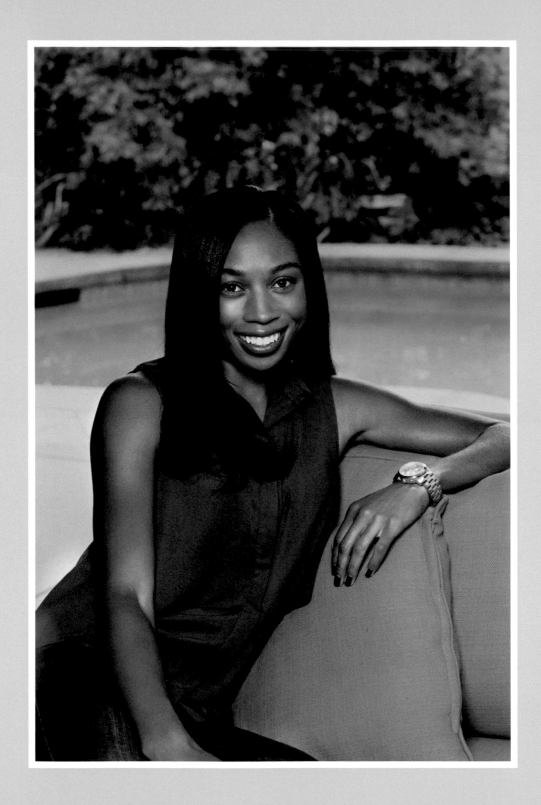

Allyson Felix

Sprinter

SKIN CARE

I'll wash my face with Olay cleanser and then use the Olay Complete lotion with sunscreen, which is great because I'm outside all day. The most important thing is keeping moisturized. After a training session, I'll do facial wipes to make sure my skin stays clean. For nighttime, it's the same routine only I use a cream. But for me, I think a healthy regimen also affects my skin. I try to drink a lot of water to keep it clear. Diet is a big part of it.

MAKEUP

I don't wear makeup when I compete. There are a ton of girls who do and look fabulous. I leave it for off the track. If I'm just going around town, I love the NARS tinted moisturizer and my Tarte palette. I actually have several palettes but I love this one which has all their bronze-y colors. Bobbi Brown has a good mascara. Then I'll use that with an eyeliner—I have so many different types.

I usually hear about products from my friends, and of course I love Sephora. I'll walk in there and walk out with a million different things.

If I'm going out, I'll play up my eyes more. For my lips, I love nudes. Sometimes, if I'm going somewhere special, I'll go for a lip color. I like the matte mauve type of colors from Urban Decay. I also have glosses by NARS and Chanel. From NARS, I have the Sixties Fan, which is a deep plum, and Risky Business, which is a shimmery raspberry.

HAIR

My hair is still in braids right now. I love different styles, although this one is very easy. I always look for styles that can handle my activity, as I work out a lot. I also love going on YouTube to try different styles. I like the advice and how-tos—you can learn anything on there.

Sometimes I'll wear my hair straight, but I'll also wear it curly. It's just a little over shoulder length right now. To maintain it, I'm using the

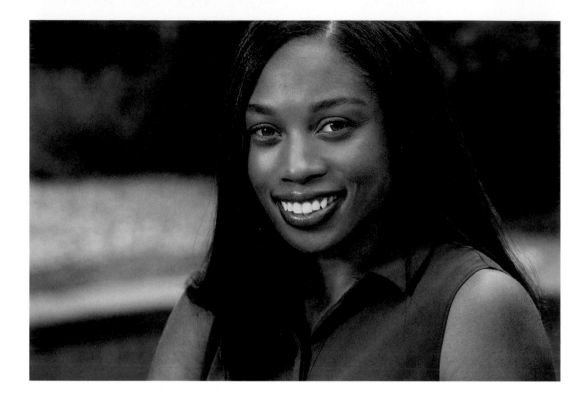

curly hair line from Pantene—the shampoo and conditioner. Pantene also has a curly hair styling custard, that's one of my go-tos.

I go to Capella salon for my cuts. I go to another place for my braids, called Mahogany Hair Revolution. It took about four hours for these braids—not crazy, but long enough! But the good part is they last a long time and you can get them touched up.

FRAGRANCE

It's a gift I get a lot. I have friends who will give me their favorites. It's a fun way to try different things. One of my favorites is Dior Pure Poison. It's great for when you're going out at night for a dinner or something like that.

OTHER SERVICES

Massage is part of my recovery process as an athlete. I see my masseuse and chiropractor every week, and on those days I get my nails done too. It's important to take care of your feet as a runner. On my fingernails, I'll have a subtle color. I'll go for a brighter pink or purple on my toes.

DIET AND FITNESS

I have to maintain a strict diet. I am very balanced. I eat a lot of fish, vegetables and fruit, and brown rice typically. If it's in-season, I'm training about six days a week. On those days, I'm typically training five hours: three hours on the track and two hours in the gym. But this is actually my off-season right now, which goes from the end of September to the end of October, so I get to splurge and let my body have a complete break. It's so important to refresh your body and your mind.

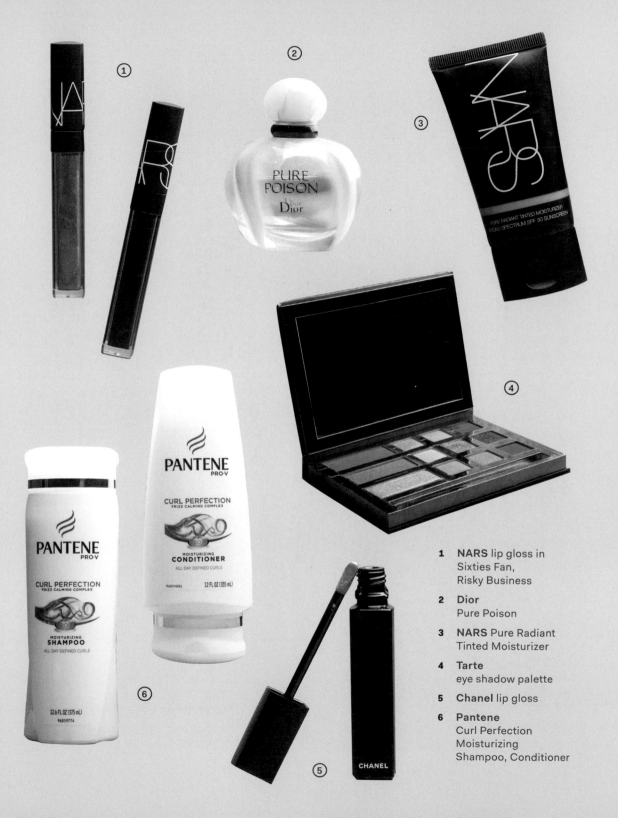

1 **NARS** lip gloss in
   Sixties Fan,
   Risky Business

2 **Dior**
   Pure Poison

3 **NARS** Pure Radiant
   Tinted Moisturizer

4 **Tarte**
   eye shadow palette

5 **Chanel** lip gloss

6 **Pantene**
   Curl Perfection
   Moisturizing
   Shampoo, Conditioner

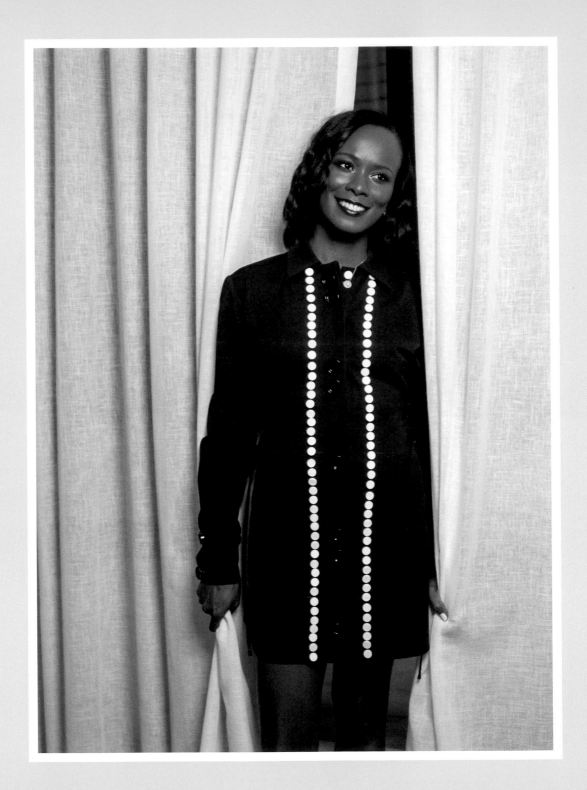

Shala Monroque

Fashion and Art Consultant

SKIN CARE

I shower in the morning and the evening. For the shower—especially since I moved back to St. Lucia—I love Dr. Bronner's peppermint bath. It's so hot most of the time right now and this really cools you down. And I just use bars of soap like Ivory.

For face wash, I'm using one by Aesop that I discovered at Barneys when I wandered in. I also got the Kiehl's Creme de Corps there. I was using Laura Mercier Ambre Vanillé Body Butter, but I wanted something with less of a scent. For face moisturizer, I use La Mer.

For night, I do the same thing. Then a few times a week, I do a scrub. I might do a cocoa butter scrub or sometimes I'll use the St. Ives Apricot Scrub for my face. And since I live on a volcanic island, I'll go to the sulfur baths. You're literally sitting in a crater, and there's mud there that you put all over your face and body. A lot of tourists come and they just put it on and wash it off. But there's a trick to it that a Rasta told me. If you go during the day, you put the mud on and you let it dry. Then after it's dried, you rub it gently so it kind of sands off and smooths your skin. It's great for detoxing and it's good for acne as well. It also relaxes you as it's really hot water.

I also have a sulfur powder because, as grown as I am, I still get hormonal acne once a month. I got it in St. Lucia, but I think it's from Guyana. It's basically sulfur and alcohol and you dab it on. It dries things up really quickly, and it's pretty natural as well. It's also good for liver spots. As a kid you'd use it, and it just makes the liver spots go away.

MAKEUP

During the day, I've been wearing zero makeup lately. It's so hot and I feel like I'm always touching my face. But at night, generally it's lipstick, blush, and some eyeliner and mascara. I just got this Nicka K lipstick at a local store back home. I like the color, Amethyst, but it feels really good on too.

I have a Chanel blush in Tweed Fuchsia and something sparkly from Armani that I use like a blush but it brightens up your face. I got both of those at the fashion shows. Sometimes you discover some really cool stuff.

I just got the foundation and powder by Black Opal. I haven't been wearing makeup at home, but then I went out with my cousin and she looked flawless. I was completely converted. Before that, I was wearing the Maybelline Mousse Foundation. I still swear by it.

Mascara, I've been using one from MAC that I really like. Eyeliner, I'm not picky. I use a mix of things. I also think it takes a while to figure out what works for you.

FRAGRANCE

Scent is a big thing for me. If I want to go back to another moment, sometimes I'll put something on to remind me. Like Prada's Amber perfume is one of my favorites. I stopped using it for a few years, but it reminds me of a certain time. I'd say now my fragrance is Seven Veils by Byredo though. A friend of mine gave it to me for my birthday about three to four years ago and I've worn it every day since. It's to the point where I can't smell it anymore. So recently I went back and got the Tom Ford Tobacco Vanille, which reminds me of Venice. I guess I wanted to cleanse my nasal palette so I can smell my Seven Veils again.

HAIR

I wash my hair only every few days. Since moving back, I cut my hair because chemical processing was really drying and thinning it out. Then I had an Afro but got bored with it, so now I'm growing it out again. Because my hair was so dry, I've gone through so many different kinds of shampoos and conditioners. Shea Moisture, which I got at Target and I'm using now, is really good. Otherwise, I try as much as possible to not blow dry or use heat. I do relax it myself, though, because otherwise it's too much trouble to deal with. If I'm not doing anything, I'll just put it in two braids or two cornrows. If I go out, I'll take them out and my hair will be wavy.

OTHER SERVICES

There's this amazing guy, Julian, who comes to my house for massages. I've been doing a lot of physical stuff—gardening and I'm building a little shack and I'm making this rock pathway, all myself—and this really helps. I moved back in with my mother, so he'll give both of us a massage, and we'll invite him for lunch sometimes.

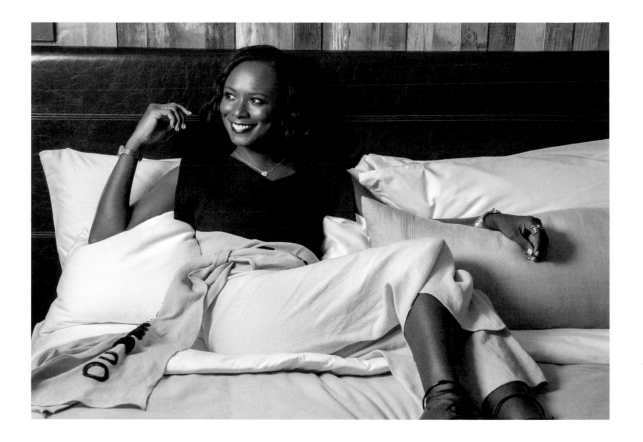

I also swear by laser hair removal for the bikini area and just any stray hairs in places you don't want to talk about. I've been going to Romeo & Juliette on 57th Street for years.

DIET AND FITNESS

I don't have a set workout. I've gotten back into shape just doing the gardening and land-scaping. Hauling rocks for the rock path is really some-thing. I also started diving. Recently, I got some sea urchin from one of my dives. I didn't realize before how many sea urchins you have to get to fill a small bowl.

Diet is not something I pay attention to. Although, since moving back, my mother has been so excited, she keeps cooking and cooking. I was like, "Stop, you're making me fat!" She does make an amazing stewed pork. Also, one of the best things in St. Lucia is that there are all these fishermen who will bring in fresh catch like lobster. Or near where I'm doing my land-scaping, there's a man who collects whelks. It's wonderful to have access to all these exotic things. He'll pass by and I'll buy a bag.

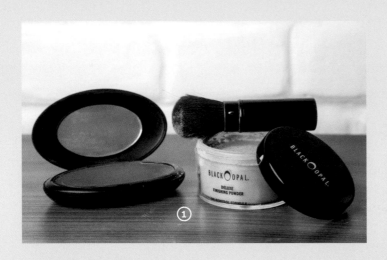

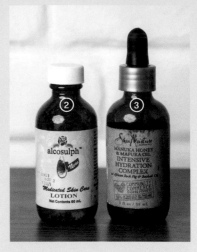

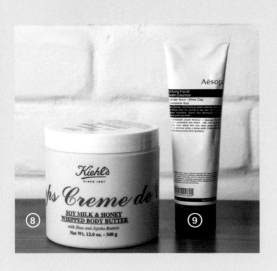

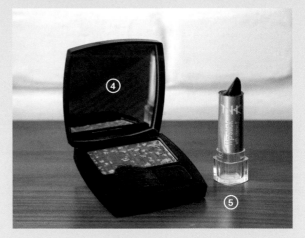

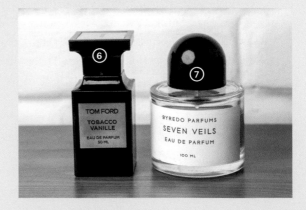

1 Black Opal
foundation, powder

2 Alcosulph
Medicated Skin Care
Lotion

3 Shea Moisture
Intensive Hydration
Complex

4 Chanel
Tweed Fuchsia Blush

5 Nicka K
Amethyst lipstick

6 Tom Ford
Tobacco Vanille
Fragrance

7 Byredo Seven Veils

8 Kiehl's
Creme de Corps

9 Aesop
Purifying Facial
Cream Cleanser

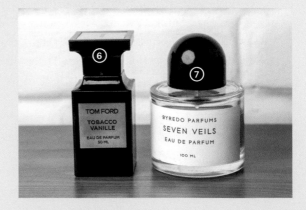

PAMELA NEAL
ON ROCK-AND-ROLL HAIR

When news broke that David Bowie passed away, I thought of Pamela Neal. The English hairstylist worked with Bowie for years and has come to define rock-and-roll hair. As St. Vincent put it, she's done basically every single cool contemporary rock star there is, including Björk, Adele, and Katy Perry. (Pamela also counts as a client the divine Tilda Swinton, who may not be a musician but has a badass aesthetic comparable to the greats.) Now based in L.A., Pamela is the art director of the established Benjamin salon, but she hasn't lost any of her irreverent spirit.

I grew up on the south coast in England in a little tourist town called Bournemouth. I always knew, strangely, that I wanted to be a hairdresser. There was never a doubt. I naturally understood how to create shape. I might have gotten some of my father's engineer brain. I probably could have created shape with anything, but everybody had hair, so I could get at it whenever I wanted to do. Surprisingly, my family and friends just let me experiment on them. The first time I cut my mom's hair, I was nine or something terrifying like that.

I didn't really think about hair as conservative or bold then. I just thought about it as literally cutting hair and creating a shape. That's before I trained. Then, naturally, as soon as I could, I got a Saturday job at a local hair salon. Shampooing

and how the salon worked was all fascinating. As soon as I was able to, I started an apprenticeship at the best possible place in town. It was the best one in town, which didn't mean it was the best in the country. It became very clear how strict the program was. The kids would go home every day crying. If you're not cut out for it, you would simply stop.

My dream was to have my own salon in some shiny city somewhere. I didn't know the editorial world existed. In the little town I grew up in, I didn't know you could do hair for magazines. All of my early influences were about David Bowie. Bowie was my guiding light the second I could remember. That's what gave me the connection to musicians in the first place. It wasn't so much that he was a musician but that he spoke the truth—his own truth. He was completely authentic to who he was. He showed me the best way is not to compromise and to just do it. He's definitely who I got my courage from, and this was from viewing him from afar.

As soon as I finished my training, I wanted that shiny city. I just knew it wasn't going to be England. England was pretty depressed and too expensive at the time. I saved up as much money as I could and got on the next plane out of town. Honestly, I saw a special on TV about Toronto and I was like, "Oh my god, that's where I'm going." And that's where I ended up. I found John Steinberg; he owned the Toronto hairdressing scene at the time. He was an original punk from London, and he had a crazy, crazy salon. Under him, I started doing much bolder work—really experimenting and with no limits. We did crazy shit. It's all about inspiration. You have to kind of really go far to cull inspiration.

My specialty eventually became cutting, but at the time, I was experimenting with everything. I was really into perms. I was setting hair on triangular blocks and pipe cleaners. Then with color, I had a vision. I knew what I wanted to see and I did it—that was thanks to David Bowie. There was also the sense of "Who cares?" I didn't know anybody, and I was encouraged by John to go as mad as possible and I did. When you experiment that wildly, nothing becomes an impossibility. So when you're on a set with Katy Perry and she needs to look like an alien or David Bowie needs to look like a lizard, you figure it out.

On working with musicians...

By then, I had made quite a few friends in Toronto. I actually met Floria Sigismondi as she was coming out of art college. I was just opening my own salon as it turned out. I followed my dream all the way.

We got together and immediately loved each other and just started experimenting. She was taking pictures and I was doing hair and makeup. Pretty soon, she was asked to do editorials for magazines, and of course I was doing hair and makeup. Makeup I knew nothing of, I just made it up. Then she started to direct as a natural progression. All of a sudden, I was doing music videos. There were big ones right off the bat, like one with Marilyn Manson, which was great in a way because we didn't know the protocol. We thought we could call the shots. We'd show up and say, "Now, we're going to make you bald and cover your eyeballs and put you on stilts. Sound good?"

Weirdly enough, people just did it. It's not like that now with all the people consulting on a video.

On working with David Bowie...

All of sudden, Floria said, "You're not going to believe this. We're going to do David Bowie." It was for a song called "Little Wonder." It was horrifying and exciting. This is the man who got me where I was without him even knowing it. I knew all his looks already.

We shot the video in New York. I had this idea, "Let's turn him into a lizard." Floria is like, "Great." When I met him, I thought I was going to spontaneously combust. I needed to impress him so badly but have him also go along with what we were proposing.

He was so taken aback. We were like, "This is what we're going to do: I'm going to airbrush some metallic lizard skin on the back of your hair and you're going to look like this and this." He was like, "Hmm ... I could try that."

As it turned out, he became my client after that until he passed away. Usually I'd see him in New York, usually at his place. Every time, I would go to the appointment thinking, "This has to be the best haircut I've ever done because he deserves the best." It's hard because he had such a wonderful witty banter. I was constantly trying to keep up with that and be clever and at the same time give him the best haircut of his life. I think he knew how I felt. I was a horror show every time.

I suppose over the years I did relax. There's a constant flood of new artists and TV shows. Sometimes he would sit me down in front of You-

Tube and show me the latest artist he had found. He was always searching for interesting people. Even his last video, he worked with someone new. He had the finger on the button—always.

Later I also worked with him on a video where he's a priest—Gary Oldman and Marion Cotillard were also in it. There was also the "The Stars (Are Out Tonight)" with Tilda, and he just looked handsome.

On working with Tilda Swinton...

Tilda was one of my clients as well, so it was funny to see them together and then giving them the similar hair and color treatment for that video.

The thing about Tilda is that it's about her face, her attitude, and her stature. She can really carry a look with no makeup and that short hair. Women of a certain age won't do that, but she couldn't look more spectacular. She's also potentially not human.

On styling Adele for the "Hello" video...

I didn't know her before. It was a fluke phone call. Xavier Dolan, who directed that video, is a genius and a celebrity in his own right. I got the call the day before the shoot. Her regular hair and makeup artist would not have time on set to do both as he usually does. Adele had a very short time to do this. So I got a very panicked phone call: "You have to come to Montreal tomorrow." Then I had to be vetted by Adele and her team. I guess I was the first who was cleared.

The look was glamorous but it was Xavier Dolan's idea of glamour. The hair was constantly moving because there was constant wind. Usu-

ally her hair is quite a solid '60s-inspired shape that generally doesn't move. This was a massive departure for her.

I really built the look for the wind. Her hair is extremely thick and straight. That was the material I had. I used a curling iron, which is not something I generally use, and then over-curled and hair-sprayed each section to keep the pieceyness and separateness of the style. When the wind went through, it would drag out her hair and create the movement I needed.

On the difference between rock-and-roll hair and "celebrity" hair...

The difference is in the attitude of the person, of course. My intention with every client of mine is to create the shape and color of the cut that suits the person in texture but also in personality. If they have more of a rock-and-roll vibe, you can push that envelope further. Hair changes are so gutsy. It's not a pair of jeans and T-shirt you can put on and take off.

That said, musicians tend to strike out on completely new ground—like Björk and Lady Gaga. I'm so in awe of that. Whereas, celebrities tend to follow what's already out there or tried or true. Tilda Swinton is an actress, but she's rare.

The other thing is that with rock-and-roll hair, there are icons of inspiration. The second you employ certain aspects, like a bleached blonde and a chopped cut, you're going to be doing Blondie. Rock icons, they last longer than just celebrity ones. They have lasting power for a reason. They were super cool and talented. Otherwise, we wouldn't still be here referencing them.

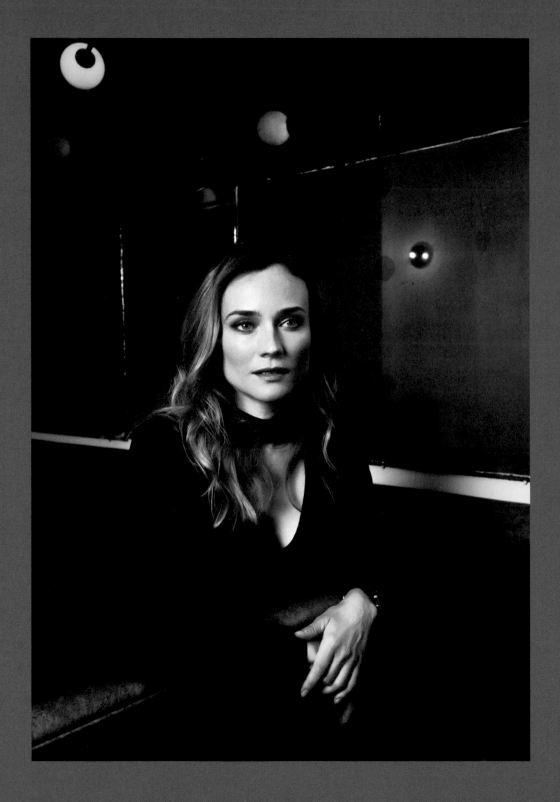

Diane Kruger

Actress

SKIN CARE

I usually start the day with this face wash from Uriage. It foams and you can find it at the French pharmacies. I've been using it for a long time—at least five years. One day I just walked into a pharmacy and started using it after a pharmacist there recommended it. Then I use a toner from Kiehl's. It's the blue one—a classic. And right now, because it's summer, I've been using the Chanel Hydra Beauty serum as my moisturizer. I always wear sunscreen. The one I'm using is also by Chanel, and it's SPF 50 but really light. For eye cream, it depends. If I use one, though usually not in the summer, it's one by Uriage. This routine works for me. I tend to break out easier, so I stick with what I've picked up over the years. I'm probably more European in my thinking because of where I grew up—the "less is more" philosophy. The sunscreen habit is from living in L.A. though—I don't like to be tan like some of the people there. And when I go to New York, all the women are so on top of it. They have their dermatologists they see for this and that. I can't keep up. I don't even pluck my brows!

But sometimes, I will do a gommage, or an exfoliating scrub, by Sensai. It's cool: It's a dry product and you put it on your face and it works. I do it once or twice a week.

MAKEUP

It depends on the state of my skin. If it's a good day, I'll just use a Clé de Peau concealer under my eyes and on any blemishes. If it's not a good day, then I do a BB cream or the Tinted Moisturizer from Laura Mercier. If I'm going out, then it's the Chanel Vita-lumière Aqua. It's interesting, because I do both American movies and French indepen-dent films—I'm currently shooting a movie in the South of France—the difference with makeup. In American movies, especially the big budget films, they definitely want the leading lady to look as good as she can. The French are always about being real or less is more; sometimes, I have to fight to cover up my pimples.

Usually though, if it's not work, I do just a brown mas-cara from the drugstore. But I always do a brow, even during the day. I use an ash color pencil by Chanel. My brows are naturally pretty thick, but I like to accentuate them with pencil because I think they give me character and frame my face. I don't need as much makeup if I do my brows.

For night, I don't like black on my eyes, but I'll usually do a dark brown liner, like a cat eye. I don't know why, but when I'm in Paris, I tend to do eyebrows and a red matte lip. I love the MAC Ruby Woo and I have a bunch of different reds from NARS.

FRAGRANCE

I wear Calvin Klein Beauty. I used to be the face of it, but I'm not anymore. I actually continued to wear it afterward. I like the idea of smelling the same for a long time. Before, I wore the Burberry scent for five years. I've been on Beauty for about six years now.

HAIR

I'm a natural blonde but it's not a very pretty blonde, so I used to get lots of highlights. Then I had to do a reddish thing for a movie a little while back, and I haven't done anything to it since. Now it's growing out and I think it's the nicest color I've ever had. The red kind of washed out and the old highlights have come through and my natural roots are out. It's darker than it usually is and I'm loving it.

For cuts and color, I have someone in Paris, David Mallett; someone in L.A., Vanessa Spaeth, who is a freelancer and is really good with blondes, especially since L.A. blondes are often too white; and in New York I go to Serge Normant.

I often use the David Mal-lett products. He has a really beautiful repair mask. I also love the Christophe Robin rose shampoo and sometimes I'll use his oil on the ends of my hair. For styling, I like the Ouai Dry Shampoo and Texturizing Hair Spray—I love the smell. And I also love Oribe products.

OTHER SERVICES

I do massages. I prefer more of a Thai massage—some-thing that's more energizing. I've tried acupuncture but just can't get into it. I'm not a spa junkie.

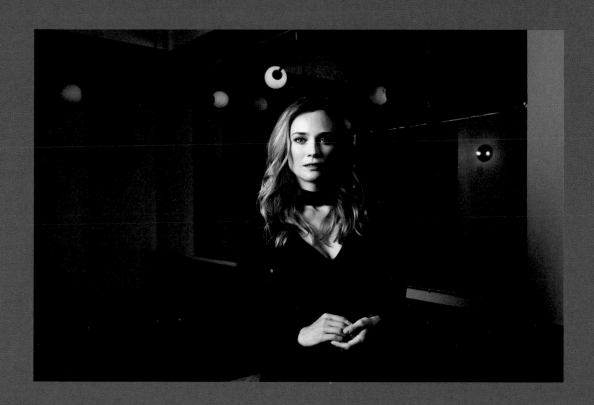
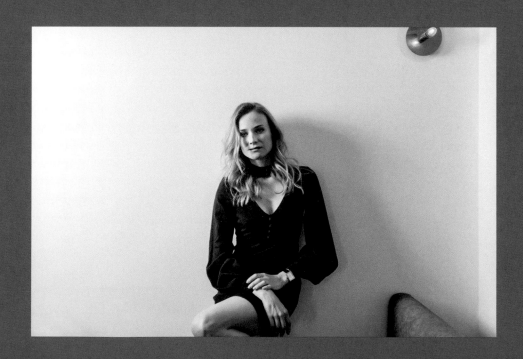

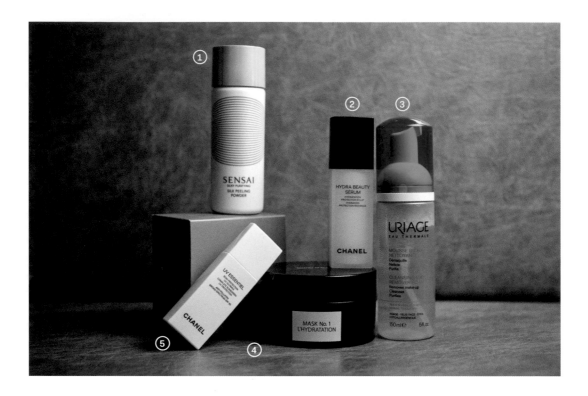

DIET AND FITNESS

I eat everything in moderation—I don't like junk food anyway—but I do exercise a lot. I probably am overdoing it. I used to be a ballet dancer, but then for years, I didn't work out. Then I got older and felt I needed to get toned and all those things, so I went to the gym. I also like to be outdoors, to cycle and hike. But now that I'm exercising, I can't just go for two or three times a week. Suddenly it's working out every day for an hour and a half. I think Paris is actually terrible for exercise. Twenty years ago when I first moved here, there was nothing. It's gotten better, but the equipment is often really old. It's harder to find good classes. But for sure L.A. and New York are fitness havens.

1 **Sensai**
Silk Peeling Powder

2 **Chanel**
Hydra Beauty Serum

3 **Uriage**
Cleansing Makeup
Remover Foam

4 **David Mallett**
Mask No. 1

5 **Chanel**
UV Essential Sunscreen

TAKING THE HIGHLIGHTING ROAD

Excellent skin care aside, highlighters have become the cure-all for tired complexions. And indeed, when chosen and applied with care, they can do wonders as a pick-me-up.

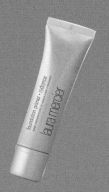 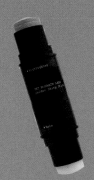 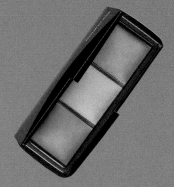 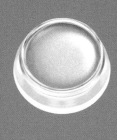

LAURA MERCIER
FOUNDATION PRIMER - RADIANCE

This easy-to-blend liquid is subtle enough to be nearly foolproof. You can wear under foundation as intended, or kick the rules for typical primer aside altogether. I dab this on the high planes of my cheeks, down the bridge of my nose, and on my browbones after I apply foundation for a hint of glow.

HOURGLASS
AMBIENT LIGHTING PALETTE

This bestseller has won over Alia Shawkat, who wears the three different luminous shades swirled together.

PAT MCGRATH
SKIN FETISH HIGHLIGHTER

A creamy stick favored by models like Lexi Boling, who says it "makes everything look dewy."

RMS LIVING LUMINIZER

Fashion designer Julie de Libran favors this coconut oil–based highlighter on an otherwise naked cheek. Another tip? "I use it under and on the sides of my eyes," she says.

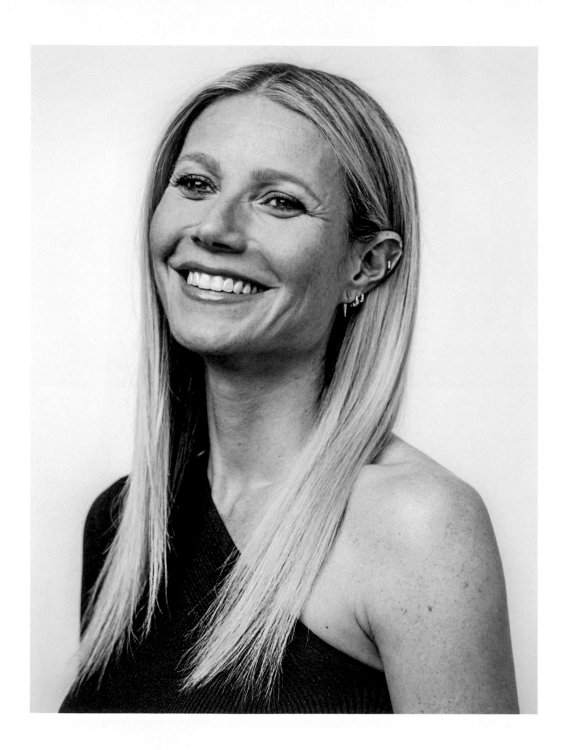

Gwyneth Paltrow

Actress and Entrepreneur

OTHER SERVICES

I'm always the guinea pig to try everything. I've got to try them all. I love acupuncture. Also, I just heard of one service called a sound bath, which might be too hippie-ish even for the likes of me. It's some new healing modality; I might have to send you in. I might not be able to handle it. But generally, I'm open to anything. I've been stung by bees. It's a thousands-of-years-old treatment called apitherapy. People use it to get rid of inflammation and scarring. It's actually pretty incredible if you research it. But yeah, it's painful. I haven't done cryotherapy yet, but I do want to try that.

SKIN CARE

I've been using my products now since I've been getting the samples back from the lab. In general, I love serums and face oils and body oils. I'm a real oil kind of girl. There's a myth that oil is not good for your skin; I don't believe in that at all.

So lately, I've been using my Instant Facial—it has some gentle fruit acids in it and you feel it go active because there's a little tingle—and seeing great results. There are also some beads in it—obviously not the plastic microbeads—and it leaves me glow-y. I think you're supposed to only use it three times a week, but I've been using it more. Then I'll use the day or night cream, or our oil, and the eye cream. Sometimes, I'll use a clarifying mask—I like this blue one by May Lindstrom. We did a big story on clean, nontoxic SPFs last summer, and there's a great one by Drunk Elephant. I also like the ones by Coola and Honest Company. I only use mineral sunscreens—never the chemicals one. I don't understand why anyone would put on carcinogens.

I also love Tammy Fender body oil—it has a lavender scent and it's smooth and really absorbs. I find oil on skin really helps the appearance. And the Organic Pharmacy has a body oil I like as well. Sometimes, I'll just use the organic coconut oil in my kitchen on my legs.

When I'm on the go, I use Ursa Major face wipes. Also, oil is really good for getting off eye makeup. You don't want to use a harsh chemical.

MAKEUP

In the day, I generally I don't wear that much makeup. The culture in L.A., you're outside a lot—there's hiking and swimming. It feels in a way that you're engaged with nature more. I usually use a little bit of Tata Harper or RMS; they each have a little cream blush for lips and cheeks. Also, Olio E Osso— it's a beautiful olive oil balm with color in it and I'll stain my cheeks with that. Juice Beauty does a great nontoxic mascara and also these liquid lip glosses. It's less and less hard to find nontoxic stuff. It's kind of amazing how much selection is available.

I often go out with just mascara and a little cheek. I don't use bronzer. You need technique to use bronzer, highlighter, and BB cream—all these things my daughter tells me about. She watches You-Tube. She's very vocal about what she likes and doesn't like. I sort of let her do her own thing at home. She loves experimenting. I obviously don't let her out of the house with a full face. But I think she's going to be way more into beauty than I am.

FRAGRANCE

I collect some fragrances, but recently my head of beauty said you have to stop wearing fragrance because it's unregulated and all that. We're having a fight about it. The problem is I think essential oils haven't mastered the art of being subtle and layered. So I'm on the fence about fragrance right now.

HAIR

I generally use Shu Uemura shampoo and conditioner. I like a lot of the Japanese ones. I have dry, damaged, bleached hair, and they work for me.

That's the one area I can't find a nontoxic product that works well. I do put the Rodin hair oil by Bob Recine on my ends. For my color, I go to Tracey Cunningham, and for cuts, I normally get a trim if I'm doing a photo shoot. The last one was with Adir [Abergel] and he cut my hair; he's amazing.

DIET AND FITNESS

I definitely believe in exercise being an important part of your routine. I'm a die-hard Tracy Anderson fan. I do boxing occasionally. I have a membership at a little boxing gym; it's pretty down and dirty.

But I have a slightly easier philosophy all around than ten years ago. I think I see now that life is really a balance, and it's great to eat nutrient-dense organic food if you can. It's also really great to drink a vodka and have French fries. Your metabolism does slow as you get older though. If I have to get into tip-top shape, I have to be more careful, but I also don't seem to care as much as I did.

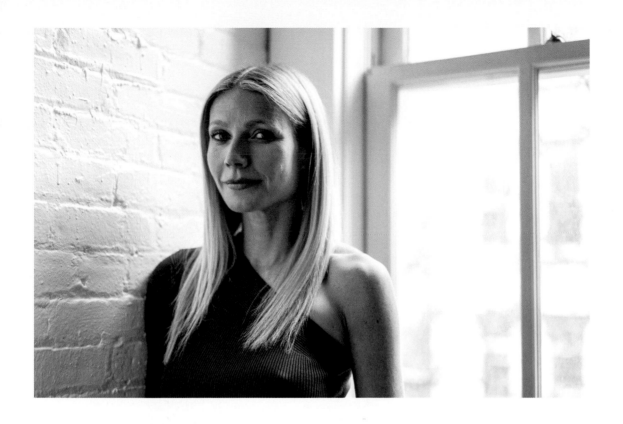

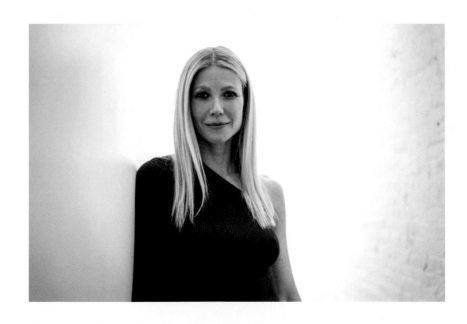

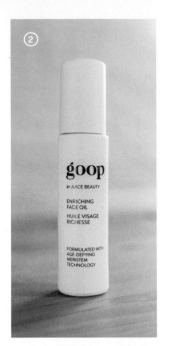

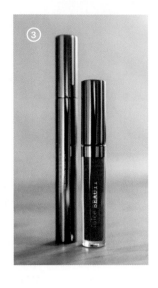

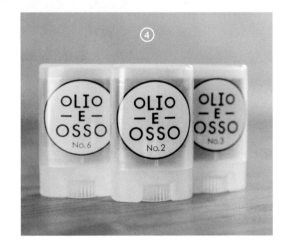

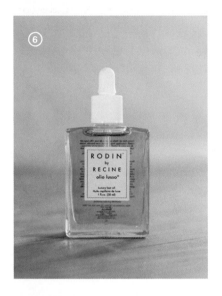

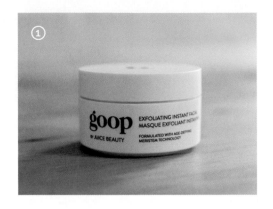

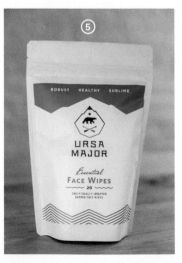

1 Goop
Exfoliating Instant
Facial

2 Goop
Enriching Face Oil

3 Juice Beauty
mascara and lip gloss

4 Olio E Osso
olive oil balm

5 Ursa Major
Essential Face Wipes

6 Rodin
Hair Oil by Bob Recine

SERGE NORMANT
ON A CAREER
IN CELEBRITY HAIR

In the celebrity hair world, Serge Normant is legendary. One look at his client list—Julia Roberts, Sarah Jessica Parker, Julianne Moore, Katy Perry, and Diane Kruger, for starters—and you'll likely find one iconic look after another that's been copied time and again in salons around the world. But among beauty editors, he's a particular favorite, because rather than come up with something that's just trendy or directional (as some famous hair stylists are wont to do), he creates cuts that truly flatter the individual without looking trite or conventional. In fact, he gave me the best haircut of my life when I was seven months pregnant with my first—who knew a haircut could lift the spirits so?

I don't know that I ever did a specific transition to "celebrity hair." I started in fashion and there never was that thought of choosing fashion over celebrity. But especially being from Paris and a child of the '60s, I dreamed of working for a glossy. I loved the photography. But perhaps the most notable shift to have happened was probably the first time I worked with Julia Roberts. We did a *Vanity Fair* shoot with Herb Ritts. That was pretty early on—it was the early '90s.

I am a hairdresser, so doing hair on a model or an actress or my mom or my friend, when I'm behind the chair, it's the same at the end of the day. But I would say I started doing more actresses after Julia.

Julia and I hit it off right away. She was shooting *The Pelican Brief* and we were in Louisiana and she had worked all night and she was very tired. François Nars was actually doing the makeup on the shoot. Marina Schiano, who was the fashion editor at the magazine at the time and who was a big model in the '60s, styled the shoot. She has a larger-than-life personality. It was a wonderful team.

Julia had shot *Pretty Woman* just a year or two before. We were all fresh and very excited. We were in an amazing location. Sometimes a place sets the tone. She was tired but so cute and sweet. I did her hair when she was almost asleep. Until today, I love those pictures. There's a very iconic one that Herb shot.

Speaking about celebrities, for me, Herb was the first to embrace them. For my generation, Richard Avedon was the dream as far as fashion photography, and he shot some celebrity shots. But Herb was the first one who had that rapport with them. He was so modern, and he lived in L.A. Working with him, François, and Marina, it was one of those great moments—whether for celebrity or fashion or not.

So that brings me to celebrity hair. To me, there's no such thing as "celebrity hair" because I never really restrict myself. I will always propose but I never impose. Forcing something on someone never works out. I may try to steer them a certain way though. For example, I worked with Sharon Stone for a long time. She had long hair and we were always joking about short hair. So when we went from long to short, we were ready for that.

Also, when I started doing more actresses, it was the '90s. There were red carpets, but celebrity hair wasn't a thing. Almost every interview I did was about the fashion shows I did. Obviously, if Julia won a big award, I would be called for interviews for that, but it was more about fashion in general.

Since then, all that has changed dramatically. I became known for doing big hair and especially on celebrities. Is that a good thing or a bad thing? I suppose you're always concerned when someone puts a sticker on you.

The truth is, I've done many simple styles and haircuts. And, of course, when we work with trends, there are strands of those trends that feel more current than others. But I've also learned to not really listen to the critics. You can't second-guess yourself all the time. When you work with a celebrity, you're working with a person and her personality. You have to remember that red-carpet hair is meant to last. There's no retouching. Those are the things that define celebrity hair I suppose.

And I'm also embracing that whole big-hair thing. When I did my product line, the second product I did is called Dream Big, which is all about volume. I thought, I might as well go for it because I like it.

Also, for me, color is very important. Color can really make or break a haircut, and it's about enhancing with the right dimension. I absolutely collaborate with my client's colorist.

Today, I get to see a variety of women. The thing I love is the strength all these women have along with the beauty and talent. With Katy Perry, I don't do her a lot, but when I do, it's so appealing to go into the music world and do something different. I've also been around long enough now to see some of these women evolve. With Diane Kruger, I used to work with her when she was a model. I look at her today and the career and person she's become—it's inspiring.

But once again, the industry is changing. It's not just celebrity anymore. There's the rise of the social media stars. I think there's always room for someone that people find interesting. For me, though, social media did not come naturally. It really took work and a lot of pushing myself to be okay with it. When you do what I do, you're trusted to be extremely discreet, and the whole social media business is about revealing things behind the scenes. It's so huge right now, there's no use fighting it. I have to embrace it.

I do have to say, and I think we can all be guilty of this, that sometimes with social media and other things on our phones, we miss the opportunity to be present in the moment. People go to dinner only to be on their phones the entire time. So I'm trying to enjoy the moment and embrace it. I've never taken my career for granted. Whether it was being on a fashion shoot or knowing some of these actresses for so long, I will never be blasé about it.

SERGE NORMANT'S TIPS FOR ACHIEVING GORGEOUS VOLUME

Starting Point

If you're talking just plain big hair, it feels dated. It feels retro. The thing is, big hair can mean so many things. It can mean just thickness. For the person at home, who looks at a fashion show and thinks, "That won't work for me," think about the one thing you can take away from it and make it work for you.

Tools and Products

That's also the approach you should take when looking at the tools and products: Find the ones that work best for you. If you have to use more than two to three products, then you are using the wrong ones. Get to know the products instead of just loading it on.

Where to Turn Up the Volume

Figure out where the volume should be that's most flattering for you. For many, it'll be the roots of the hair, but maybe for others it's mid-length volume that's most flattering.

Learn to Love Your Hair

If you really look deep enough, you'll find something to love. Maybe you don't love your frizz or curls, but you like that you have a lot of hair. Try to take advantage of that with your cut and styling.

Volume in a Pinch

Spritz a texturizer at your roots and all over your hair. Put your hair upside down and do a very loose bun on top of your head. Do your makeup while it sets. Then let it loose and you'll have a tousled look with some kind of volume. Alternatively, part your hair in the middle and twist each side of your hair into Princess Leia buns. Spritz with texturizer, set, and let go.

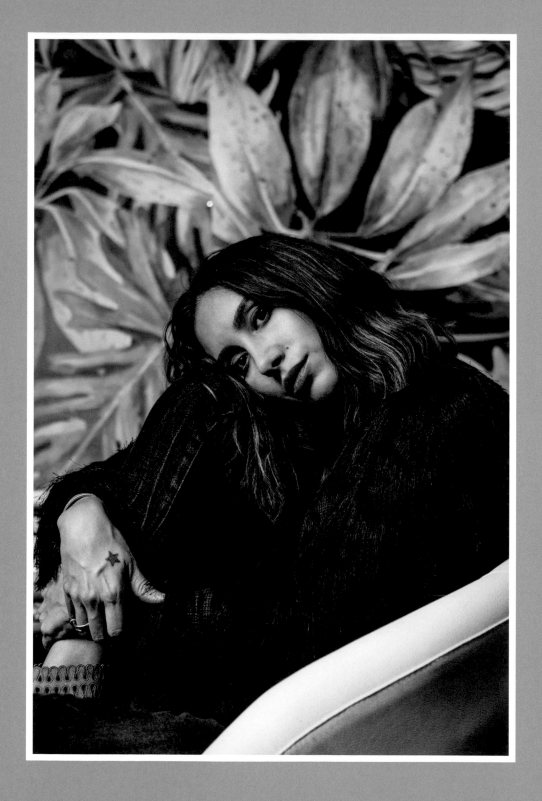

Jen Atkin

Hairstylist and Founder

of Ouai Haircare

SKIN CARE

When I wake up, I usually make English Breakfast tea, a Dr. Lipman shake, and then try to get a quick workout in before I start my meetings and emails. Then I use the same products for day and night. I wash with AyurMedic orange blossom scrub. I like the Active Serum and a Hydra-Cool Serum by Clinical Innovative Skincare. Every other day, I use retinol, which is so good. I also use the Dr. Dennis Gross pads once a week. It's a routine I got from my facialist, Shani Darden. If I need it for night, I'll use the Honest Beauty Makeup Remover Wipes. And during the day, I'll wear Epionce SPF 30 daily under my makeup. I'm also traveling a lot and then I have a bunch I take with me. I love the Charlotte Tilbury Goddess Skin Clay Mask, SK-II sheet masks, Glossier Balm Dotcom, and Clean & Clear Oil Absorbing Sheets. The Tatcha hydrating mist is also great for flights.

MAKEUP

I usually do my makeup in the car as I am always on the go. I use Kiss EZ Trio Lashes and a dash of Hoola Benefit bronzer and the Tarte x Hrush eyeshadow palette. For mascara, I use one by Fiona Stiles and then the Troy Surratt liquid liner. For lips, it's either the Lorac lipstick in Flower Child or Kylie Cosmetics Lip Kit in Kristen. For brows, they've been such a thing lately. I get them shaped by Anastasia then lightly fill them with her pencil and swipe Glossier Boy Brow for hold.

Otherwise, I don't feel like I always need to be "photo ready." That's what a pretty filter and Dr. Ourian are for!

I definitely like to put on more makeup—like contour, highlight, and extra lashes—if I'm going out at night. The Glossier Haloscope highlighter is really good. I also have always loved Sade growing up, and her red lip is a huge inspiration for me. I think that once you reach a certain age, you find your "look," and mine is a cat eye with a red lip. I like to look a bit Spanish.

I've learned so much by working with such talented makeup artists like Joyce Bonelli, Mary Phillips, Mario Dedivanovic, and Hrush. I wouldn't know a thing about contour if it wasn't for them.

HAIR

My hair is naturally dark brown and wavy. I usually get a Brazilian blowout by Anthony French at Andy Lecompte Salon to control the frizz and

wave pattern. Then I'll go to Cassondra Kaeding at Sally Hershberger for chocolate-brown color to add dimension. For cut, Gregory Russell, Renato Campora, or Kevin Murphy usually cuts it. I like to keep it in a piece-y bob that hits right around the shoulders.

If I had to pick one product, I couldn't live without my Ouai Wave Spray. I literally use it before almost every blow dry to add volume and texture, and I love spraying it in my own hair for a natural wave. I also love the Christophe Robin Volumizing Mist and Kevin Murphy's powder duster, and of course the Dyson Supersonic Hair Dryer.

FRAGRANCE

I love the Juliette Has a Gun fragrance Another Oud for the musky scent. I discovered it from my travels in the Middle East. All the women there smell so good.

OTHER SERVICES

I love getting massages at The NOW in L.A., which is a

massage boutique. I also love Silk Day Spa in NYC, and Ban Sabaï in Paris. When in L.A., I get my nails done at Olive & June.

DIET AND FITNESS

Khloe Kardashian and Jenna Dewan Tatum have really inspired me to get my work out on. I recently did a Danskin shoot with Jenna and had to hit the gym immediately after. I've been obsessed with ClassPass for Pilates Plus and Barry's Bootcamp workouts. I love that they offer classes throughout the day so I can squeeze something in with my crazy schedule. I always bring my workout clothes with me when I travel and try to go to a Barry's class or hit the hotel gym.

I try to eat healthy most of the time, but when you're traveling and on set, it's hard to be consistent. I usually do a Dr. Lipman cleanse a couple times a year to reset my system though.

①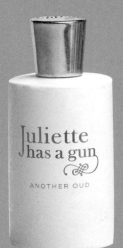

②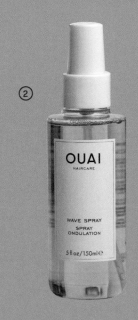

③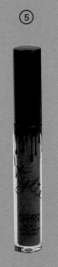

④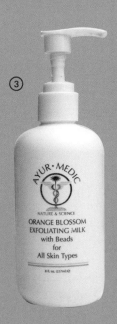

⑤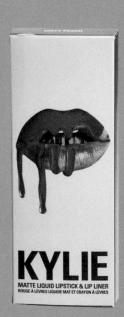

⑥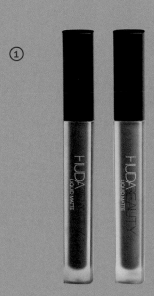

1 **Huda Beauty**
Liquid Matte Lipstick

2 **Ouai**
Wave Spray

3 **AyurMedic**
Orange Blossom
Exfoliating Milk

4 **Dyson**
Supersonic Hair
Dryer

5 **Kylie Cosmetics**
Lip Kit Kristen

6 **Juliette Has a Gun**
Another Oud

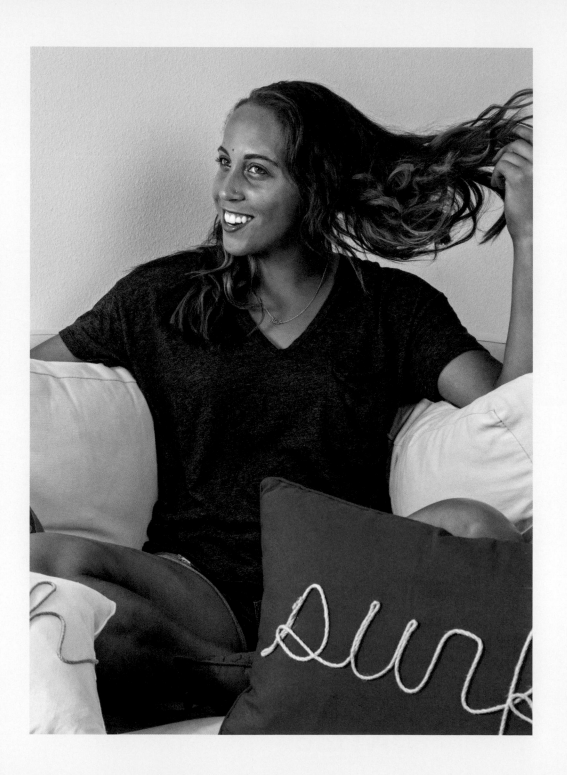

Madison Keys

Tennis Player

SKIN CARE

Since I practice early in the morning most days, I wake up and wash my face with Clean & Clear Morning Burst. I only use it in the morning and I feel like it actually does wake me up a bit. Then the first thing I put on is sunscreen. I try to do it within fifteen minutes of waking up so I'm protected by the time I'm out the door. I use the Neutrogena oil-free sport formula for the face. For the body, I'll use the Neutrogena Wet Skin spray. I try to get at least SPF 50 on me.

After practice, I use the Evian face mist, which is great because it helps clean your face and it refreshes you. I like it after working out and on the plane. I'll, of course, hit the shower. I am obsessed with the Bath and Body Works Warm Vanilla Sugar line. Someone gave it to me when I was fourteen and I've been using it ever since. I use the sugar scrub and body wash and lotion. Sometimes, when you get older you think maybe you should grow out of certain products and try something else, but I still really like it.

I use moisturizer only at night—philosophy's Hope in a Jar. I tried the line's Miracle Worker undereye cream a while back and I fell in love with it. When I needed a moisturizer, I went back to the brand. Also, two or three times a week,

I'll do a Caudalie face mask. It's a purifying one because I have combination skin and I'm sweating so often it can be really tough to keep clear skin. Especially if you're wearing a visor or something like that, it's just sitting on your head and you'll break out all underneath. It can be a disaster.

MAKEUP

I have pretty even skin tone naturally, but being out in the sun all the time, I'll get red cheeks and a red nose and maybe one part of my skin is darker than another. I don't like heavy foundation, but if I use something tinted, it helps blend everything together. I've been using Urban Decay One & Done. It has primer, SPF, and a tint in it.

I use Benefit They're Real! mascara. For eyeshadows, since I travel so much, I love the Urban Decay Naked palette because it has so many colors all right there. Then I use the Urban Decay setting spray. It's so good. Otherwise, living in Florida, you'll go outside for twenty minutes

and realize, "Oh, my mascara is sliding off my face."

For eyeliner, I use the Urban Decay 24/7 pencils. I use black or brown most of the time, but if I'm going out, I like to use purple because it sets off my green eyes. I'll use the eyeliner on my water line and then use a matching eyeshadow to go over it a bit. Then I'll use the shadow as a liner on top.

I tend not to wear blush, but I do love highlighter—Benefit Watt's Up. If I'm going out, I'll put some on my nose, my cupid's bow, under my brows, and on my cheekbones.

I've always been more of an eye person, but recently I've been really getting into lip colors. I like the Tarte matte lip stains. They travel so well and stay all day. If I want my lips to be shiny, I'll just add Victoria's Secret clear lip gloss on top.

Before, I'd say all my beauty stuff came from trial and error at Sephora and hearing from friends, but now I'm on Instagram a lot. The videos are so great—there are so many different makeup artists doing

looks and you can see exactly what it's going to look like on someone with the same skin tone—and they're why I've been so into lip color now. Sometimes, I'll just go in my "Explore" page and look for makeup videos, but I follow @WakeUpAndMakeup mostly.

FRAGRANCE

When I was at the Australian Open this year, one of our player gifts was a department store voucher. I wanted a new fragrance; the one I was using, I didn't like anymore. The second I tried Giorgio Armani Sì, I loved it. I've been using it for six or seven months now. I don't love a super sweet-smelling perfume, but I also don't like when there's too much of that musky smell. This one is just a really good combination of the two.

HAIR

It's usually straight up into a bun when I wake up. There's not much to do in the morn-

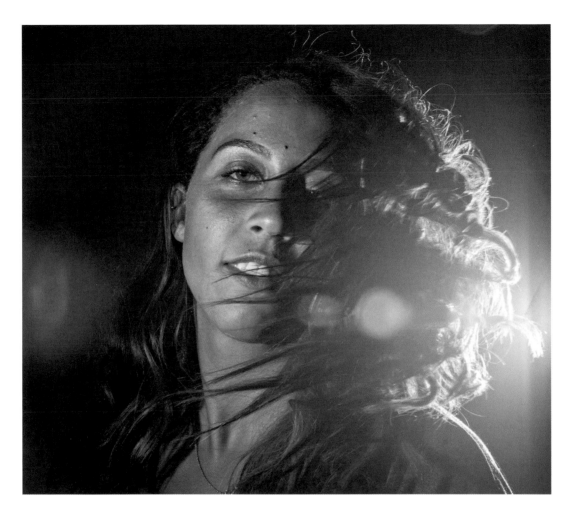

ing. But at the end of the day, I'll let it down. I have naturally really curly hair. Every girl who has really curly hair fights it at some point and tries to make it as straight as possible. But over the last year, I'm way more open to wearing it natural and I'm loving it. I use the Bumble and bumble curly hair line. That's shampoo, conditioner, and styling. I also do a lot of moisturizing. I'm constantly in the sun and my hair is pulled back tight, so there's so much breakage. Sometimes, I'll just leave the conditioner in for an entire day. I also love putting in coconut oil.

I had a horrible experience once when I wanted an inch or two off and the stylist didn't listen and cut three and a half inches off. That was a little traumatizing, and I've been trying to grow it out. Otherwise, I recently got my hair cut and colored at a place in Bettendorf, Iowa—where

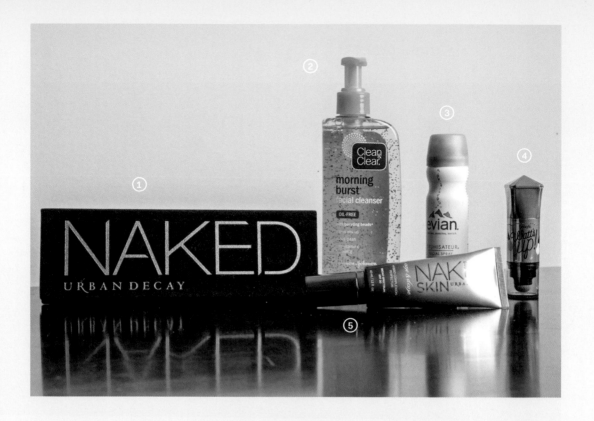

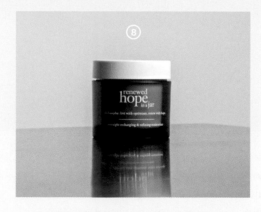

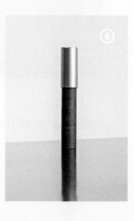

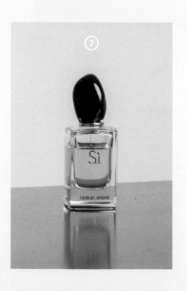

1. **Urban Decay** Naked eyeshadow palette

2. **Clean & Clear** Morning Burst

3. **Evian** Facial Spray

4. **Benefit** Watt's Up

5. **Urban Decay** Naked Skin One & Done

6. **Tarte** Matte Lip Tint

7. **Giorgio Armani** Sì

8. **philosophy** Renewed Hope in a Jar

I grew up. It's called Haus of Heir. They opened maybe like two years ago, and I was really looking for someone who understood my curly hair.

My natural hair color is a really, really dark brown. Right now, it's dark at the roots but I wanted to go a little lighter for summer, so there are some blonde pieces—like balayage.

OTHER SERVICES

I get manicures and pedicures every two weeks. For my manicures, I get gel. Colors, I usually go with black and dark purple, but sometimes I'll do a navy. I really like Lincoln Park After Dark by OPI or the House Blues color as well.

I have a physical therapist who travels with me. He's a chiropractor actually, but he also does acupuncture, so I get acupuncture almost every day. This has been going on since last November. I've had lots of injuries and it really hindered my playing, so I had to take that extra step to hire somebody. I actually hate needles, but this doesn't hurt. It's really interesting how one day

it can be used to treat muscle soreness, and another day it can be used for relaxation and it'll put me right to sleep.

DIET AND FITNESS

Being a tennis player, our toughest part of training is the off-season. It's not the longest off-season—we're usually done the first week of November, we'll have a week or two off, and then we have six weeks before our first tournament— that's when we're doing tons of tough fitness: maybe two to three hours in the gym and not being on the court as much. Obviously as you get closer to the tournaments, you spend more time on the court. Right now, I'm spending about two and a half to three hours on the court every day. Also, for me, I have the mental practice side to my game. I have someone I call and talk to at least once a week. We talk about what's working and what's not. She's great at giving me tools to work it out.

I obviously have to eat pretty healthy to stay in good shape, but for me, a big part of

my diet is letting myself have that occasional dessert. I have a huge sweet tooth. My favorite is Ben & Jerry's Half Baked Ice Cream. But I also have to watch it. I'm actually lactose intolerant, so sometimes I'll do the Ben and Jerry's lactose-free line. There are a surprisingly good amount of lactose-free options out there now.

DR. DENNIS GROSS:
HOW TO MAINTAIN CLEAR SKIN FOR AN ACTIVE LIFESTYLE

Call it the fitness revolution, but most women I know incorporate some kind of workout into their weekly routines. This phenomenon has created an incredible lifestyle change, but our skin care regimens likely have yet to catch up. For how we adjust to these new skin care conditions, I sought out New York dermatologist Dennis Gross, M.D. He's a fountain of technical knowledge—he created a bestselling peel for his eponymous line by balancing a trio of different acids, after all—and he's terrific at dishing it straight.

Wash Your Face.
That's the first thing. It's something that's so fundamental, but you'd be surprised. People will go to bed with makeup on. Athletes might wait a couple hours after working out before washing. It's even important to wash your face before a morning workout. Your night moisturizer may contain oils or lipids that will actually start to settle into pores and impede the secretion of sweat during your workout.

Skip the Makeup.
People will often workout with makeup on. But here's why you need to take it off before you hit the gym: Makeup will get into your pores and enlarge them because of the build-up. So much so that even routine washing will become inadequate.

Choose Oil-Free Sunscreen.
Sunscreen is a must, and it's preferable to use oil-free sunscreen. For the same reason you need to wash off your nighttime moisturizer, you don't want any stuff that will clog you up.

Battle Bacne by Choosing Cotton.
If you start breaking out on your chest or back, you should get to it early. If you can, you need to wash off any moisturizer you've put there, especially if you perspire a lot. Another thing, and some might think it's radical, is you should revert back to cotton clothing. There's been this whole movement to wear "wicking" clothing. But the whole idea of clothes that wick spawned from not wanting to

walk around with a wet T-shirt after a workout, not because the sweat somehow magically evaporates. What happens is that the perspiration stays on your skin and it's not absorbed into the clothing. Cotton will absorb the perspiration. If you don't want to walk around after a workout with a wet tee, then you can layer a cotton T-shirt under a "wicking" one.

Exfoliate Regularly.

It depends on your skin type whether daily or weekly, but you should do a regular routine here. It's not only deep-cleaning—it can get at deeply embedded makeup—but it's also anti-aging, which is especially good for outdoor enthusiasts with sun damage.

Consider Adding Vitamin C to Your Routine.

If your workout takes you outdoors, the sun can cause uneven skin tones or sun spots. I love vitamin C here. It's very effective at evening out skin color and also building up collagen.

Build Up Collagen Now.

It's best to prevent problems and get to any concern as soon as possible. Sunscreen can only do so much. And don't underestimate what the sun is doing to your collagen, which is what gives your skin tone. It's not just about sun spots. There's vitamin C that can improve and stimulate collagen, but retinol also works. In the office, there are lasers that can firm and stimulate as well. The more you mix up your methods, the more dimensionality you can preserve. Don't just bank on one method.

Incorporate Low-Impact Workouts.

If you're a lifelong runner, every time your foot hits the pavement, it vibrates through your skin—so it impacts your collagen. I don't recommend doing only activity that hits the pavement; it really jostles the collagen. If you're a jogger, then also do elliptical.

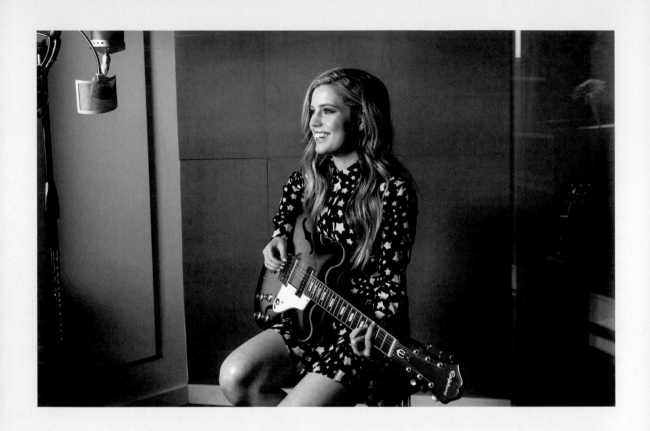

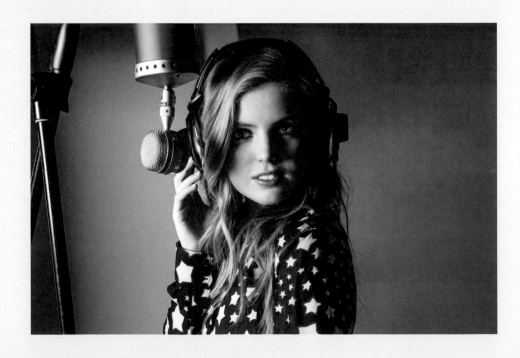

Sydney Sierota

Musician

SKIN CARE

I wash my face with a Kombucha Cleanser by Scientific Organics. Then I use this mist with bee propolis by Epicuren, and then their probiotic face cream. At the beginning of the year, I was breaking out, and that's when I started going to a facialist at Touch of Faith Aesthetics. That's where I got all these product recommendations. They said to do this routine every morning and night; it's made the biggest difference. I was weirded out for a second with the Kombucha Cleanser. My brother was actually obsessed with drinking kombucha for a while, so I was familiar with it but only as something you consume. But hey, if it's good for your body, it could be good for your face?

For travel or taking off makeup, I use Yes to Cucumbers face wipes because I have super sensitive skin. Any other wipe makes me red. For spots, I use Ultraluxe Drying Potion. I found the lotion when I started to break out; I started asking all my friends what they did. My friend Chloë Moretz actually turned me on to the lotion. Her skin is amazing.

Sometimes, I'll also use this face mask from Epicuren that you leave on for five minutes and then you rub it off and it exfoliates your face. It comes in a little blue bottle, and it really does the trick for clearing up clogged pores.

MAKEUP

I use a tinted sunscreen with SPF 30 by a brand called Sun Si'belle. I use that as my makeup base. Then I use the NARS Radiant Creamy Concealer around my eyes. I was looking at Instagram and seeing that this makeup artist Hung Vanngo—I love what he does—was using it. Then my makeup artist at home started buying it too. I'm generally fair-skinned, so I'm always using the lightest color of concealer and powder. Sometimes, the product is not even light enough. I'm the only one here who doesn't have the glowing tan skin. But I have the glowing white skin!

Then I'll use bronzer and highlighter for my face. I use the MAC Mineralize Skinfinish as my normal powder, and I use just a darker shade for the bronzer. The highlighter I use is a mix of the Hourglass Ambient Lighting Palette with the

Laura Mercier illuminating one. The funny thing about highlighting is everybody my age is doing it and knows the three areas to highlight, whereas my mom didn't do any of that growing up.

I always do a kind of bronze-y smoky eye, even for daytime. I love the Tom Ford Cocoa Mirage palette. It's so good for everything and really easy to build on. Then I do the Tom Ford liner in Metallic Mink and smudge it a bit. The best mascara is L'Oréal Telescopic. It's dark and easy and looks good on everyone.

I don't put blush on every day. But if I do, I use Tom Ford in Frantic Pink. The Tom Ford stuff is a recent thing. My viewpoint—and I think probably a lot of people my age too—is that we're up for trying any product. I'm coming from an open-minded place. I just want the end game to happen. I just want the great skin and good beauty products.

HAIR

Right now I'm in the middle of transitioning to blonde. My natural color is like an ashy brown that will sometimes get highlights in the summer. It's also curly and dry. It's a lot to deal with. Looking at my old photos, my hair looks pretty wrecked. I've found a way to get it under control. Every time after I wash my hair—I use Paul Mitchell—I use a mask by Kevin Murphy. Chloë also turned me onto that. She's got it all figured out!

As for my blonde, I'm actually getting it done again tonight. It's about slowly adding more and more highlights. My boyfriend's dad owns a salon in San Diego and that's where I go. He's been doing my hair for about a year and a half. It's called the Hair Zone. And his mom does nails. It's a girl's dream!

FRAGRANCE

I go between a couple different ones. The main one I use now, I actually created. My neighbor owns this little shop in L.A. called KleanSpa, and you're able to go there and make your own perfume or candle. I'm obsessed with vanilla. I did two different types of vanilla and then added a hint of tobacco and some orange blossom. I was going to leave for Europe and see Stonehenge at the time, so I called it Sweet Stonehenge. It's kind of silly but it's also a nice memory.

The other one I like is by Mary-Kate and Ashley Olsen—Elizabeth and James Nirvana Black, the one you can get at Sephora.

OTHER SERVICES

I usually get my nails done in L.A. by this cool Japanese woman, Yoco. Her Instagram is @leafa_nails. I was at Chloë's house and she was doing nails and that's how I started using her. She can do any design. If I'm going to get my nails done, I might as well go for something fun. Right now two of them are a marble design. It's really cool and the other three are white with a couple jewels. Sometimes I'll do a ton of jewels on just one finger. I like a variety but to still have the designs go with whatever I'm doing.

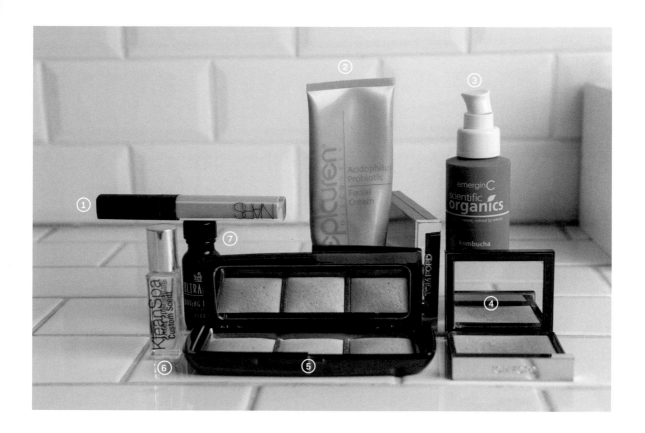

DIET AND FITNESS

For six years, I was gluten-free, soy-free, dairy-free. I had allergies that forced me to eat healthy. But recently I got tested again and I wasn't allergic to any of them anymore. Your body changes a lot. But I do try to stay really healthy. It affects my performance. I do yogurt with granola in the morning, a chicken sandwich for lunch, and a pretty simple dinner—I love sushi.

I started working out three years ago. I was thinking, "I'm close to becoming an adult. I might as well try it out." I started with yoga. Then, I branched out to Pilates, and I'll do that three times a week. I try to walk a lot, but in L.A., there's often nowhere to walk to. I also do the BBG [Bikini Body Guide] program—it's an ebook and also an app. The woman is from Australia, and her workouts are only twenty-eight minutes. It's awesome when you're traveling.

1. **NARS**
   Radiant Creamy Concealer

2. **Epicuren**
   Acidophilus Probiotic Facial Cream

3. **Scientific Organics**
   Kombucha Cleanser

4. **Tom Ford**
   Frantic Pink Blush

5. **Hourglass**
   Ambient Lighting Palette

6. **KleanSpa**
   Sweet Stonehenge

7. **Ultraluxe**
   Drying Potion

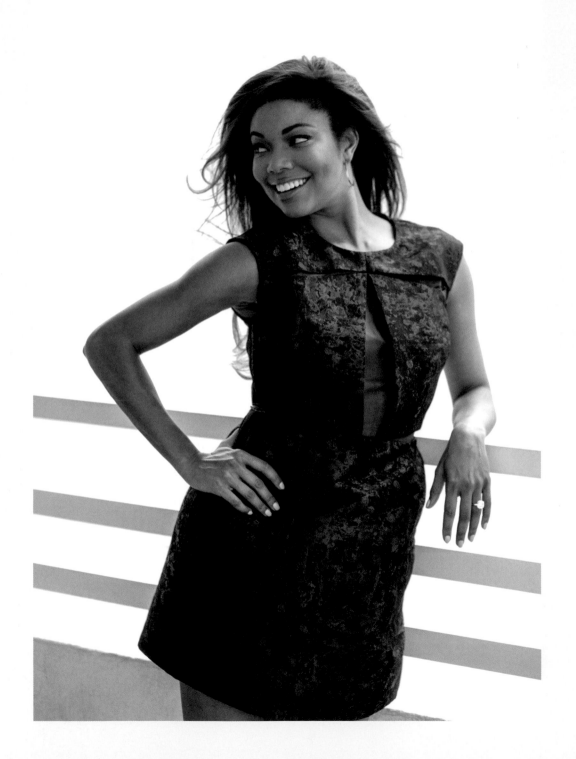

Gabrielle Union-Wade

Actress

SKIN CARE

The first step on my beauty and wellness path starts with water. I try to drink a gallon a day, and I try to get thirty-two ounces in with breakfast. It's the biggest thing for hair, skin, nails. And I'm filming *Being Mary Jane* in Atlanta now and it's hot as hell here. Then to the shower: I use a pink grapefruit face wash by Neutrogena—I'm a spokesperson for the brand—and Rainbath shower gel. I'll finish a warm shower with a really cold rinse. It refreshes my skin and improves tone and circulation. After, I tend to use oil for my body.

For my face, I keep it old school. This week, we're on nights, so sleep is sort of hard to come by. I've had puffiness. I chill some tea bags—right now it's Lipton—and use them on my undereye. Lately, I've been going through a hormonal shift and getting blemishes. My saving grace has been the Rapid Tone Repair, which helps fade dark marks.

During the day, I keep an Evian spray bottle on set, just to give a blast of cool. I'm also a huge lip balm girl. My summer lip chap situation can be a little extreme, and I have a home-made trick to moisturize on the plane. I figured out how to make a home scrub with brown sugar and olive oil, and I use that to exfoliate my lips. I keep a little container of it in my purse.

MAKEUP

If I'm not working, I don't generally wear a lot. Luck-ily, I kind of like my face. I'm pretty much a lip balm, eyeliner, and mascara girl. The trick to mascara is to use a little vibrating motion with your hand to give a thicker application. If I want drama, but not a whole face, I might smudge the eyeliner with a Q-tip for a smoky look. I keep the rest of my skin bare, so you're strangely mysterious yet fresh-faced.

For nighttime or events, it's generally somebody else doing it. But if left to my own recourse, I'll pump up the smokiness. For my wedding, though, I'm for soft and pretty. I'm not a big fan of people experimenting with beauty for weddings. Then they come down the aisle looking like strangers. Fortunately, or unfortunately, I've been on a lot of red carpets. I can't really reinvent the wheel with a hair-style I haven't tried before. I'm not going to do a wacky bun. I'm going to look like the best version of myself possible.

FRAGRANCE

I have a signature fragrance: Lumière Noire. I wear it every day, all day. With perfume and deodorant, I don't mess around. Especially working in the South in extreme heat, the likelihood you'll end up smelling is very high. How I discovered the scent: My girl-friend, who owns a boutique in Miami, started carrying it. But it took me a minute. Let me go home with this free sample and see what the mis-ter thinks. When I walked into the bedroom, he said, "What is that? You smell amazing." So that was it. It's probably been about a year and a half now.

I've also found some really cool products here on my days off. I kind of love this one: I AM Love Chakra Crystal Mist. The label says you're supposed to set your intention with it for the day—don't lose your mind and become a psychotic actor—so I've incorporated it into my routine in the morn-ing. It's kind of like my last little exclamation point to my beauty routine. After I get out of the shower, I walk through this mist of pink rose feeling like Donna Summer.

HAIR

I work with Larry Sims, a hair genius and innovator. He also works with Lupita Nyong'o— he did her hair for the Oscars. Actually, he's on set with *Being Mary Jane,* so I'm especially lucky. Larry and I met a long time ago, when I was filming *Bring It On.* He started as a background dancer with Missy Elliott and the singing group Blaque. He segued into hairstyling and started under Ken Paves.

When I'm not working and I can't get to the salon, I do my own deep conditioning treatment. In *Finally Famous,*

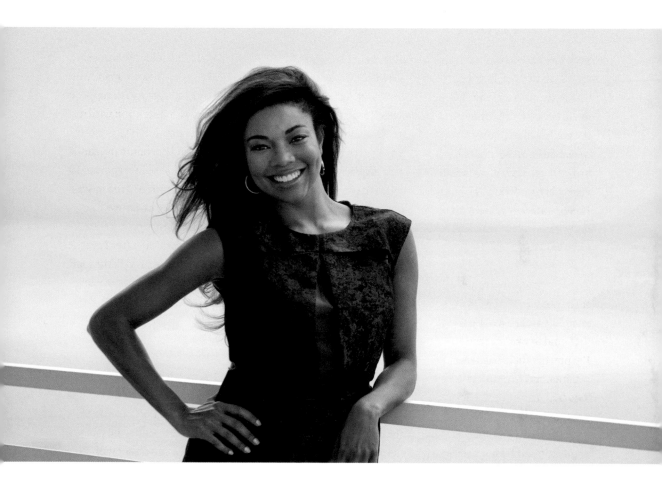

it was a role that took me blonde. It was a strange and fascinating experience with very interesting reactions. Suddenly my character and integrity were questioned. It took a lot of time to lighten and lift, and ultimately, when the movie was over, my hair fell out. I spent the last year trying to get it back to healthy. I have a hooded dryer at home. I put on conditioner —Carol's Daughter has a great repairing mask—put on one of those cheapie hotel shower caps, turn on *Downton Abbey,* and sit under the dryer. When I'm styling my hair, I'll blow dry it and prep my edges—anyone with coarser hair texture, there's an amazing invention by Madam C. J. Walker that you use along the edges of your hairline. Then I'll flat-iron.

SERVICES

I swear by massages every week. With manis and pedis, I get gels—obsessed with Gelish—and go every two weeks to change the color. I also love a good facial. For a lot of us women, every month you go through a crazy hormone situation, so at least once a month, I treat myself when I feel bloated and unattractive. I might still be bloated afterward, but I try to make myself cute. And I started getting acupuncture from this great guy in Miami—James Rohr. Dwyane was getting it for migraines. He suffered from them for many years and it was debilitating. I saw how much it really helped him and thought, "Hey, I have a host of ailments." For me, going from day to night shoots, you can get insomnia. It's helped me with that. I'll go a couple times a week if I can.

DIET AND FITNESS

I didn't pay attention to diet and fitness until magazines and blogs started with the super zoom images. As if that's not enough, they'll draw a circle with an arrow pointing out the exact imperfection. I try to stay active. When I'm working, I'll get Freshology meal delivery. Right now, in Atlanta filming, I work with an Earthcandy Arts chef who does vegan, gluten-free, etc. I became vegan Monday through Friday. What I want might be biscuits covered in gravy, but unfortunately, I have to stay the same size for work from beginning to end.

When I'm not working, I try to be reasonable. One day maybe it's a bacon cheeseburger, and another day it's quinoa and kale. I try to stay close to my fighting weight so when it's time to go back to work, I don't have to do one of those crazy diets.

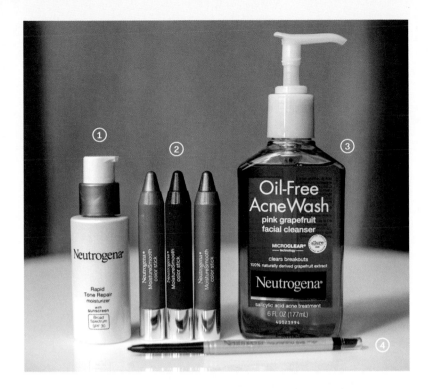

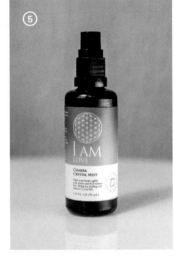

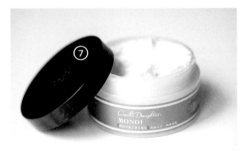

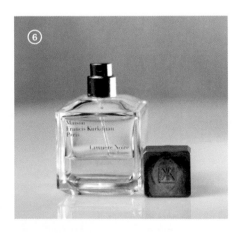

1 **Neutrogena**
Rapid Tone Repair

2 **Neutrogena**
MoistureSmooth
Color Stick

3 **Neutrogena**
Pink Grapefruit
Oil-Free Acne Wash

4 **Neutrogena**
Nourishing Eye Liner

5 **I AM**
Love Chakra
Crystal Mist

6 **Maison Francis
Kurkdjian Paris**
Lumière Noire

7 **Carol's Daughter**
Monoi Repairing
Hair Mask

DENDY ENGELMAN
THE NEW METHODS OF ACHIEVING CELEBRITY SKIN

Manhattan dermatologist Dendy Engelman, M.D., is one of my go-to resources for new developments in skin care. She keeps up with cutting-edge research, but perhaps best of all, she's able to break down complicated technologies and science-y jargon into understandable concepts. Plus, she has a Southern charm thing (she's from South Carolina) that's a pleasure to interact with, especially in the hustle-bustle of a New York day. Probably her celebrity clients, like Sofía Vergara, might say the same thing. They also go to her for her work, which is subtle in all the right ways— that is, undetectable.

Everyone will tell you the idea of good celebrity skin changed with high definition cameras, and it's true. Before, the cameras were more forgiving. Now you have to look perfect, from every pore and every angle.

With this new standard of perfection, I hear women say that the celebrity look is impossible. They say they're genetically blessed. But it's not true. What they're doing is they are aging better because they are doing a significant amount of small procedures that add up over time instead of a one-time overhaul.

Filler and Botox

In the last five or six years, patients have started focusing on every single fine line. That's a major shift from the classic places that filler and Botox were being used—places like the frown lines between the brows and crow's feet. Now filler is being used in tons of tiny places, like the little lines at the ear crease or the tiniest little pore indentation between the eyes. Because of the demand that HD puts on the celebrity, the patient has become intolerant to the smallest imperfections.

Another change that has happened: Before, it was more about using filler and Botox, but now it's mainly filler. Technology has advanced. We didn't have fillers that we could put in the upper face before. That changed with the introduction of Restylane Silk and Belotero. They are very subtle, and it's almost like using an airbrushing filter if you use them correctly.

Lasers and Skin Texture

If you're talking about a celebrity, before, it was difficult to tackle texture issues because celebrities don't have much time to be down and out of the spotlight. The lasers were effective when they were introduced, but harsh. It was the classic '90s red, red face. You would need to coordinate between shoots and movies and arranging for separate entrances for them to sneak them in and out.

Laser medicine has significantly changed and actually even changes every month. Before, the laser just blasted the skin; now the lasers have really sophisticated fractionation. That means the lasers are only causing injury to some of the cells in the treated area. That allows the skin to heal faster—think of a light scrape versus a whole area being completely injured. The downtime now is much more tolerable. It has also reduced the risk of pigmentation disorders.

Body

This is an area that celebrities pay a lot of attention to but perhaps the average woman does not. So many of them are doing scantily clothed scenes or bikini scenes. They're doing lymphatic massage. If there's a problem area, they all have their own trainers and chefs. They are human though; they have problem areas that are tough to diet away. The other thing is all the trends on the red carpet. On top of the movie, they have to promote it and often in low-cut dresses. There's nowhere to hide a thing anymore.

I often use lasers like Fraxel on the back, chest, and back of the hand. The one thing I notice when I see a red carpet is how perfect the top stars look, not just in their faces but the skin on their bodies. If you look at Jennifer Lawrence when she first came out, for example, and then see her today on the red carpet, you'll notice the difference is in the skin on her body. The top stars, the skin on their bodies looks practically airbrushed now. You really have to be perfect from head to toe.

The chest, particularly, is a giveaway as we age. The skin is actually thinner there and prone to more creasing. That's something patients who have done a ton to their faces might forget about. You don't want the skin between your face and your chest to have a disconnect. When applying creams and SPFs, you have to think of your neck as part of your face. The same thing goes for the skin on the back of the hand.

The chest, also as you age, may start to have lines. I might do filler here and there. I might recommend a silicone sleep pad for side sleepers. If you're a side sleeper now, you might gain chest wrinkles over time simply from the gravity of being in that position.

Fillers might also be used to touch up the back of the hand and even the crease above the knee for those who say their knees look old.

For the underarm, I might use Exilis, which does ultrasound and radiofrequency. It tightens the place up. I had a patient yesterday who wanted it done right in front of the bra, that part that might bulge out a bit. She's on camera. All these women are worried about aging themselves out of jobs. They are up against people twenty years younger than them, and they're being shot in Hi-Def. Some people might fault them for being vain, but this is part of their careers.

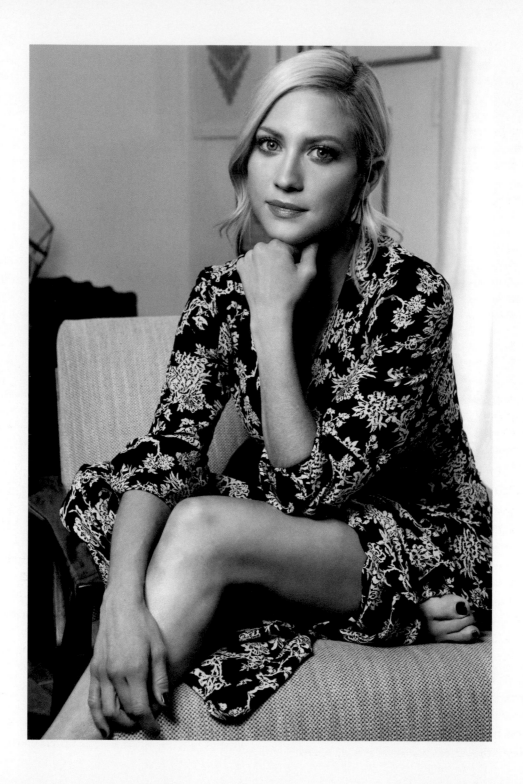

Brittany Snow

Actress

SKIN CARE

I go to a dermatologist named Christie Kidd. I grew up with pretty problematic skin. I actually am prescribed her Clean Natural Facial Cleanser. It's basically coconut oil and tea tree oil and chamomile. And then I use these things called Fresh Pads afterward. They're not really prescription, but it's just through her office. Sometimes I'll use apple cider vinegar as a toner. Everything is natural. I'm pretty specific about going natural with my skin. I go to a facialist—Amy Rae Aesthetics. She wants me to use all natural products. So I use coconut oil to remove my makeup and Vaseline to take off any unwanted things around my eyes. I use basic natural sunscreen with no added chemicals. It's the most basic Olay sunscreen—it's cheap and from the drugstore and nothing crazy in there.

The natural beauty thing is something I got caught into later, once I heard about how your skin is the biggest organ in your body. I think you start to think about that around age thirty. You start looking at your face a little differently. You can't be eating and drinking whatever you want—not even for diet or weight reasons, but because you can see it in your face.

MAKEUP

I use L'Oréal foundation, but I only use a little bit. I mostly use Laura Mercier Secret Camouflage concealer. I use it on my trouble spots and underneath my eyes. I do use bronzer, because I'm super pale. I like the Hoola bronzer by Benefit, and I use normal Maybelline Great Lash mascara. It's just the best and it's cheap and everyone knows about it. I pretty much do my entire makeup in five minutes.

I am obsessed with lipstick and lip glosses. I collect them but I probably don't use them enough. It's because I love makeup packaging. My favorite thing to do is to get makeup and unwrap it. I have every type of lipstick. And I'll have all my lipsticks out in my bathroom. It's almost like a display. It's just pretty to have Chanel around. It sounds really silly, but when I bought my house, my bathroom was kind of my favorite part. There's a lot of room to put things on display. It also makes me more Zen to have things out.

I never used to care about brows until the past couple of years, but now everybody is super into them. I'm playing this person on *Crazy Ex-Girlfriend* who is this crazy brow artist. I'm watching all these tutorials online for the role and I've been trying them out, which is kind of fun. My guy friends and I always have this discussion. My best guy friend was saying, "I just don't understand the eyebrow thing." Women go crazy with them. The Anastasia pencil, that's what I usually use. It's pretty light and the color is similar to my eyebrow. I don't like to go too dark.

The funny thing is my eyebrows are naturally curly (my hair is naturally curly) and it's interesting when people are shaping my eyebrows and will point them out. I'm like, I know.

The thing about beauty that has changed for me is that I'm less influenced by the standards of the industry now. It was a benefit to start working in the industry so young, but it was also detrimental to grow up around people and things that were so beauty focused. I was so aware of what I looked like and what people thought about me. But then I grew out of it, and only just recently, I've stopped stressing about it. There are so many other things to think about. I can't tell you the last time I opened the beauty section of a magazine.

HAIR

I don't even know what my natural color is anymore. I think I've been every single color. One of my favorite things to do is to change my hair color. I really like to see what happens and what clothes I can wear and what roles I can play. I maybe change the color every four to six months. My natural is probably a light blonde-brown maybe. That's what I had as a kid. I don't even know what color is most comfortable for me. Maybe red. But my mom really doesn't like it. The thing with hair color is that it can be an interesting study of people to see how they react to it. I just lightened it to the lightest blonde I've ever had, and it's definitely changed the way people treat me. My hair colorist and stylist, Rick Henry, is a really good friend of mine. I've been going to him since I was nineteen. Because of all the coloring, I do a lot of keratin masks. I'm a big fan of masks, and, when in doubt, I put one on when I'm watching TV. I love Kérastase; I'm a big fan of their masks and oils. And I'm a big fan of putting coconut oil in my hair. Sometimes I just put that on or olive oil. The hard part is getting it all out.

FRAGRANCE

I'm pretty particular about it. I don't like many things. I had a boyfriend once who said I smelled like his mother—it was awful. I had no idea that could

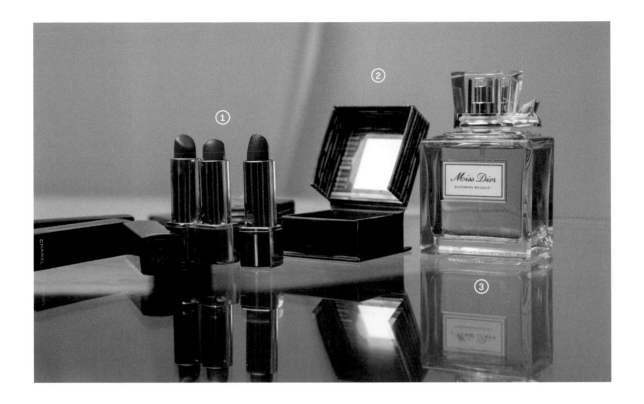

stir up so many feelings. I wear Miss Dior, which I love. It's light and young and really fresh.

OTHER SERVICES

I go to Amy Rae for facials and then I get massages and acupuncture there. It's my one-stop shop. There's a nutritionist that also prescribes me supplements. She assesses from a holistic perspective what you're missing.

DIET AND FITNESS

I wish I could be 100 percent vegan, but I would never say I was. I respect people who are, but for me, I try to be as much as I can. I used to eat a lot of artificial things back when I was a kid. I used to drink Diet Coke and have Splenda. In the past years, I've cut all of that out. I feel so much better.

I do Pilates at WundaBar three times a week; I love the reformer machine. I also go to SoulCycle twice a week. My roommate and I love to run. Last year, when I used to live by the beach, I was doing really well. Now, we don't do our six-mile runs. But we try.

1 **Chanel**
lipsticks

2 **Benefit**
Hoola Bronzer

3 **Dior**
Miss Dior

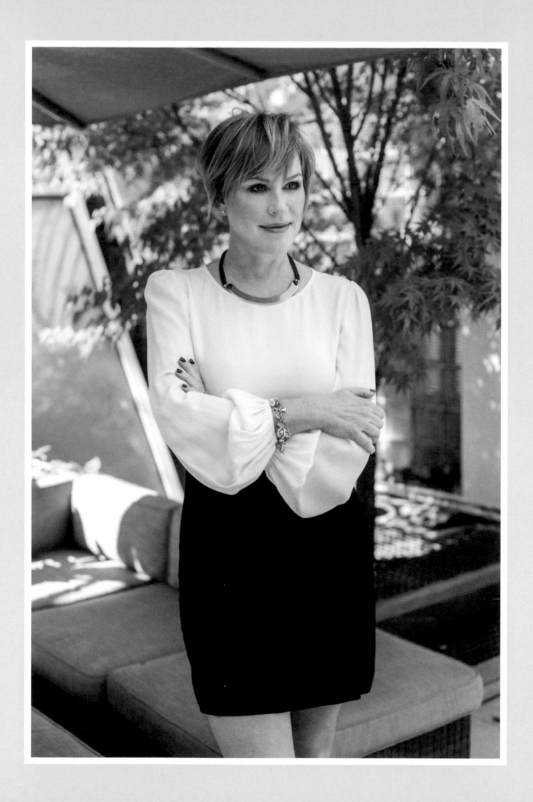

Molly Ringwald

Actress, Musician, and Author

SKIN CARE

I use these products by Kim Sevy, an aesthetician that I met in New York through this really great dermatologist, Dr. David Colbert. Well, she ended up leaving New York and going to Utah and developed her own skin care line; it's called Alkim Me. There are these steps and things that come in vials and packets. The first one I use is a mist and then a vitamin C serum. You actually get that in a vial and mix it yourself so it stays really strong and potent. The third is a hyaluronic acid and the fourth is an oil elixir. These products saved my life. I was traveling all the time and staying in hotels and using their products. My skin was going crazy. Now I use this day and night, and if I really have an issue, I'll go to Colbert and he'll sort it out.

Otherwise, I'm a shower in the morning kind of person. I use Dove soap. But I'm also a bath person. I just moved from California to the East Coast. In California, I wasn't taking any baths because of the drought. Now I'm relieved! Sometimes I'll take baths with my little kids, or if it's just me, I'll do one at night. I use Epsom salts if I'm exercising a lot.

MAKEUP

When I'm not working, I wear almost no makeup. I feel like I put all my concentration and focus on my skin: If your skin looks good, then you don't have to wear a lot of makeup. As a teenager, I wore so much makeup because I was always trying to cover up my freckles. Now I like my freckles. I might use a little concealer: I'm still a big fan of the YSL Touche Éclat. And I really like Laura Mercier reflecting powder. Also, I always put on sunscreen. For years, I was always on the hunt for the perfect red lipstick and now I'm on the hunt for the perfect sunscreen. It's like the holy grail: finding something that works but one that doesn't clog your skin. Right now, I really like this tinted one by Eve Lom. It doesn't feel mask-y. I'll even wear it out at night.

For eye shadows, I use the Naked palette by Urban Decay. It's great for travel because it's got everything in there. I stick with mattes and taupe-y colors; I don't really like shimmer that much because it accentuates every little fold. At this stage of my life, it's not helping a lot. I may put a bit of liquid liner on the lash line—Stila has a really good one. If I'm going somewhere, I'm a big fan of the '60s Jean Seberg *Breathless* black wing-tip liner.

I do love lashes. I wasn't blessed with great lashes, so very often, if I'm going out, I'll wear fake ones. I'm pretty good at applying them myself, and the best ones—I like Ardell—you can just pick up at the pharmacy. Unless I'm performing—if I'm doing a jazz performance, I'll go for a smokier eye—I don't like it when the strip goes all the way across. It irritates my eye. There's also this Korean makeup store in Los Angeles and they have an amazing stock of lashes too. Whenever I'm there, I'll buy a whole bag of lashes and stock up.

I'm not super picky about eyebrows. I'll usually just use a brush and then some powder—whatever is lying around. Right now, I'm using Anastasia Beverly Hills, but it depends what hair color I'm at. I've been blonde the past couple of years. When my hair is red, it's really hard. I think people sometimes tend to use red pencils with red hair and it always looks bad. I would go with something a bit more taupe-y or caramel. It doesn't match exactly.

For cheeks, I've been using a cream blush from La Prairie. The makeup artist used it on me for *Jem and the Holograms*, and it was really nice. But I tend to use something for a while and then move on to something else.

My lipstick is Make Up For Ever in #42. It's a great red. That's my secret weapon when I'm on stage. For just everyday though, I like to do a more natural look. I've been gravitating to Josie Maran lip stain in Coral.

FRAGRANCE

I wear Carthusia Corallium. There's actually a funny story behind it. I got married in Italy about seven to eight years ago, and my husband and I honeymooned in Capri. We went into a store and the salesperson there told me Carthusia

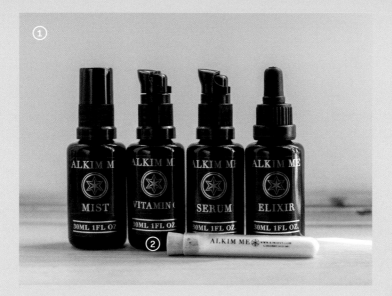

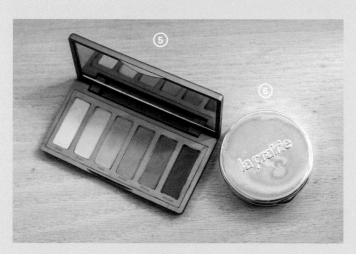

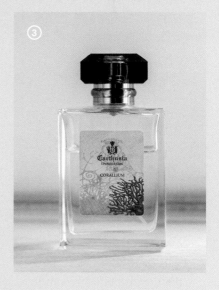

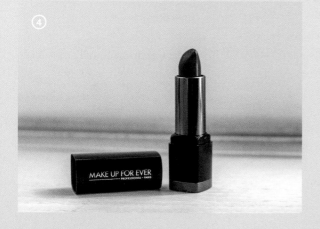

1 **Alkim Me**
Mist, Vitamin C,
Serum, Elixir

2 **Alkim Me**
Vitamin C powder

3 **Carthusia**
Corallium

4 **Make Up For Ever**
#42 lipstick

5 **Urban Decay**
Naked eyeshadow
palette

6 **La Prairie**
Cream Blush

wasn't found anywhere but there. He totally sold me. Then I was in New York and found it at [C.O.] Bigelow. I'm so gullible!

HAIR

I'm not sure exactly what my hair color is right now, and I'm not totally sure I love it. My hair has gone back and forth: It was really blonde, then it was red, and then I had to go back to blonde for reshooting scenes for *Jem*. Then I decided I wanted to go back to my natural color, which is reddish brown, but my ends have the old color. For products, I'm very partial to Oribe. I use the Signature Moisture Hair Masque. I use Oribe shampoo too, and the Oribe Royal Blowout spray. A hairdresser used the line on me a while ago and I just loved it. I'm really picky about fragrance and I love the smell.

When I visit the hairdresser, I have them put in Olaplex. It's a chemical that they can put in with the bleach that strengthens your hair. I want to grow out my hair. Right now, it's around earlobe length and my goal is shoulder length. The Olaplex helps; I feel like all the colorists are using it now.

OTHER SERVICES

I usually do nails but I'm giving my nails a break right now and just getting them buffed. I'm working on how to play the ukulele too, so I have to keep my nails really short.

I definitely get massages when I can. There's a guy in New York who works on all the Broadway people. His name is Greg Miele. He's the person they call when the star twists an ankle and needs rehab. Actually, I wouldn't say it's massage as it is very intense bodywork.

DIET AND FITNESS

For exercise, my two favorites are yoga and running. I had a person in L.A. for yoga, but I'm actually looking for someone in New York. I like yoga that's more athletic, so more Ashtanga than Iyengar.

For food, my motto is to eat as healthfully as I can and to eat only food and not food products. But I'm a serious foodie, so I'll never be the person who cuts out carbs completely. I never want to say goodbye to gluten. I'm sure I could probably weigh less than I do if I was more regimented, but then I wouldn't have the life I do. I love the social aspect of eating and going out for meals. My philosophy is just to enjoy life.

POWER LIPS

Call it the power of red, but women have long relied on the scarlet hue to create signature looks.

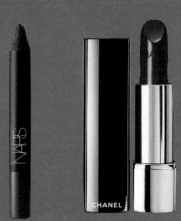 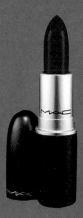 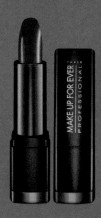 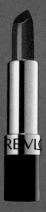

NARS CRUELLA

This warm red is a favorite of Charli XCX ("When I was younger, I was quite scared of a red lip, but then I started listening to French '60s Yé-yé pop," the pop star says) and Zoë Kravitz, who mixes it with NARS Dragon Girl for the perfect shade.

CHANEL ROUGE ALLURE IN 99-PIRATE

Isabel Toledo swears by this tube. "It's almost a uniform now, and it just makes you look sexy," she says.

MAC RUBY WOO

When in Paris, Diane Kruger pairs this matte red lip with strong brows for a spare yet impactful look. Priyanka Chopra is also a fan.

MAKE UP FOR EVER ROUGE ARTIST INTENSE IN #42

Molly Ringwald loves this vermillion hue with satin finish. When she's performing jazz onstage, it's her "secret weapon," she says.

REVLON CHERRIES IN THE SNOW

"My mother wears it; I wear it. I've worn it for a very, very long time—red lips have become my signature," says Patricia Clarkson.

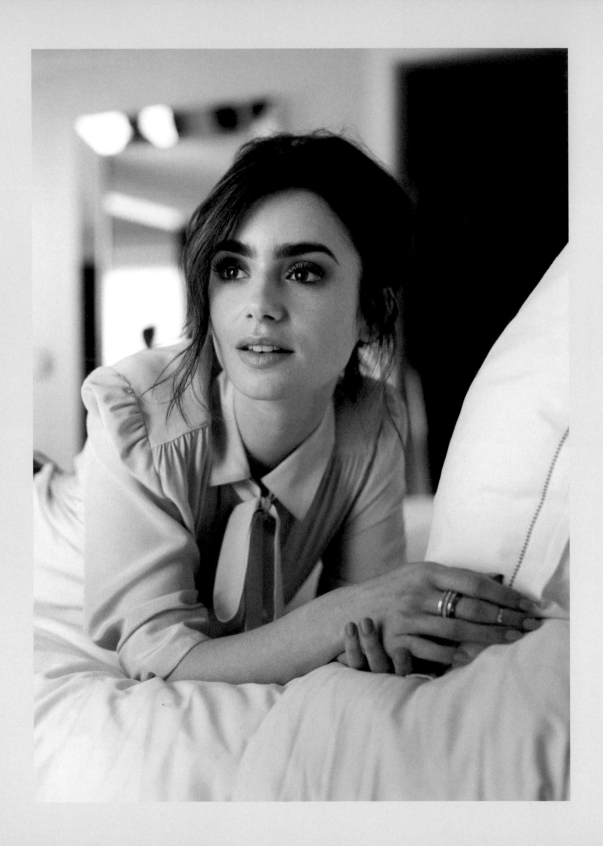

Lily Collins

Actress

MAKEUP

When I'm off duty, I wear very little. My motto is the less there is on you, the less there is to go wrong. If I am wearing makeup, I love the Giorgio Armani Maestro Glow. It's so luminous. And it lets my freckles still shine through. If I need it, I'll do the Armani powder too. The important thing, especially in L.A., is that nothing looks coated on. You've got the sun and pollution already, so you don't want more stuff clogging you up.

Then, I always do a swipe of mascara. I grew up being obsessed with the Hypnôse Drama mascara. I'm very thankful the whole big brow look is an "in" thing right now. I'm like, "Everybody keep embracing them!" They do need to be tamed on occasion. I use the clear Great Lash mascara from Maybelline for that.

I always wear lip balm. I love Smith's Rosebud Salve. I'm constantly reapplying.

If I'm going out, I might throw on a tiny bit of blush and a lip. I really love the YSL lip colors. I'll go for a deep plum. It just works with my pale complexion and dark hair. It may take me a while to apply it and get it perfect. I'm no makeup genius.

SKIN CARE

First, I splash cold water on my face just to wake me up. And then I use the Lancôme Énergie de Vie line. I'm an ambassador for the brand, so I've tested all the products. These are the ones that work for me because I feel like they brighten and the finishes aren't sticky. I use the facial wash, the toner gel, and a cream.

Then, I always put on a sunscreen. There's no California tan about me. People assume that I can't tan, but I actually can. I went on a trip to Hawaii when I was younger and came back so tan that people were like, "What happened?" It's just not something I actively do. I want to embrace my ivory. I've been using a Kiehl's sunscreen which is super light and doesn't have a fragrance.

During the day, I'm constantly reapplying hand cream. My grandma used to do it all the time, so maybe I got it from her. I love the smell of rose, and there's a hand cream by Crabtree & Evelyn with a rosewater scent that I have with me everywhere. It's so silky, and it makes your cuticles look amazing.

For night, I do the same process, but depending on how dry my skin is, I might do one of the Génefique by Lancôme masks. If I'm feeling dry, I'll also put liquid coconut oil on my body. I just get it at Whole Foods.

One thing I like to do, morning or night, is putting mint or spearmint oil on my temples and the back of my neck. There's this aromatherapy quality of both easing tension and waking you up. I have one by Saje that's called Peppermint Halo. It's an insanely incredible product. It comes in a rollerball and you put it around the edge of your face. It makes your skin feel like it's on fire and is cooling at the same time.

HAIR

I've kind of lost track of what my natural color is. I just got back to brown from my watermelon red hair. That was for a role: I was shooting a movie in Korea, and my character's name is Red. It's nice to be back to brown because I know the makeup colors that work. But my hair has been through so much. There's the coloring, but I've also been doing a lot of period pieces lately and they're always curling my hair. Kérastase, I've used the products forever. I use the Bain de Force line, which is for repairing and reconstructing. If I want extra volume, I'll use some of the Shu Uemura Fiber Lift gel. If I've gone a couple days not washing it, I'm the biggest fan of the Oribe hair sprays, whether it's the beach spray or the dry shampoo spray. For me, it's not easy to do hair, so if I get it done by a pro, I'm always trying to save the hairstyle.

FRAGRANCE

There are three scents I gravitate toward. There's rose, and also I've seen bergamot in a lot of the things I like. The other one is oud. Growing up, I was always drawn to deeper smells more than the super feminine ones. When I dabble in essential oils, I like a mix of all three. Many I get from wandering the aisles at Whole Foods. But when I travel, I love to go to apothecaries. When I was in Korea, there were some amazing stores. Or I'll go to Abbot Kinney in Venice and there are wonderful little boutiques there. Basically, I have the biggest array of oils and hand creams. Some people are obsessed with shoes and bags; I'm obsessed with my little collection.

OTHER SERVICES

I have always loved massages, and hot stone massages are one of my favorites. Ever since I was little, my dad used to stay at The Peninsula in L.A., and I kind of grew up knowing

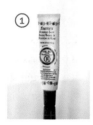

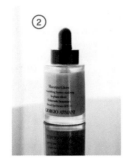

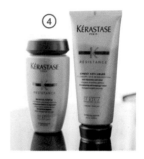

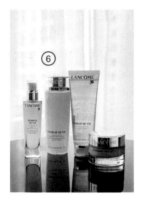

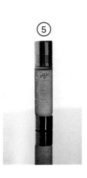

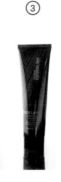

1   **Smith's**
Rosebud Salve

2   **Giorgio Armani**
Maestro Glow

3   **Shu Uemura**
Fiber Lift gel

4   **Kérastase**
Bain de Force line

5   **Saje**
Peppermint Halo

6   **Lancôme**
Énergie de Vie line

everyone there. I started going back for the spa. I always ask for my girl Jessica. I'm also fascinated with how beauty and skin care is treated in other countries. I had a really incredible experience when I was in Taiwan. It was my last day, and my friend and I had extra time. We went to this house where they treat you on the floor. They wash your feet, and there was an amazing massage, and then we had tea.

DIET AND FITNESS

I've always loved being active and I used to do sports—basketball, soccer, volleyball—growing up. Now I love running, biking, and swimming. I also go to these dance cardio classes at Body by Simone. The trainers are so empowering there—it doesn't matter if you can't dance well.

During the day, if I'm hungry, I eat something. I've always been a very healthy eater. In England, it was basically eating at the farm. It was bangers and mash, of course, but it was very much about fresh, healthy food. Then living in L.A., it's an ideal place for that. I don't eat red meat. I'm big on chicken, fish, and vegetables. It's a way of life for me. I don't think about it as a diet.

Acknowledgments

As any writer knows, the final word, and frankly any number of words, would not have been possible but for the many wonderful people behind the scenes and along the way. Having written for many editors in my career, I know the value of Anita Leclerc, my editor at *The New York Times Style* section, whose superb wit, elegant editing, and supreme sense of style is the stuff writers dream of. My many thanks as well to my colleagues at the *Times* who have shared stories and contacts, to Alex Ward, the *New York Times* book editor, and to my fellow beauty junkie Holly Dolce, my editor at Abrams, who made this book happen in the first place. And where would I be without my family, who, to put it mildly, puts up with me. My sister Grace Chang brings me back down to earth when I get overwhelmed with beauty hype. A heartfelt thanks to my nanny Celine Elva for being wonderful, responsible, and loving with my babies when I wasn't able to be there. My husband and best friend Ronen Shapiro has been my guinea pig on more than one occasion. And to our girls, Ellis and Sky Shapiro, who have often reminded me that while products are nice, there are few things more beautiful in life than waking up to a gurgle of laughter.

aging, 80, *172–73*, 227, *238–9*
Atkin, Jen, 216, 216–9

Boling, Lexi, *73*, 164–7, *207*
Bonet, Lisa, 152–6, 155
Botox, 4, *172–3*, *238*
bronzer, 16, 50, 89, 130, 160, 162, 217, 229, 241, 243
Brown, Bobbi, 128–33, 133

Charli XCX, 144–7, *249*
Chopra, Priyanka, 19, 134–7
Clarkson, Patricia, *73*–7, *249*
Collins, Lily, *19*, 250–3
colorists, *12*–3, 16, *33*, 102, 124, 157, 242
concealer, 58, 72, 84, 120, 125, 127, 153–4, 160, 169, 182–3, 204, 229, 231, 241, 246
contouring, 162–63

de Libran, Julie, 100, 100–3, *109*, 207
dermatologists, *33*, 123, 226–7, *238–9*
diet and fitness, 10, 17, 24, 31, 39, 43, 47, 53, 61, 64, 68–69, 77, 83–4, 92, 98–9, 102–3, 105–6, 112–3, 121, 126, 133, 136, 142, 146, 150, 155, 160–1, 166, 178, 182, 189, 192, 197, 206, 210, 218, 225, 231, 236, 243, 248, 253
Diggins, Skylar, *109*, 140–3
Dobrev, Nina, 48–53, 49, 52, 109
Dormer, Natalie, 180–3
Dubreuil, Laure Heriard, 62–5, *157*

Ellis Brooklyn, 5
eye cream, 7, 15, 57–8, 67, 90, 106, 113, 136–7, 159, 161, 203, 209, 221
eyebrows, 8, 17, 36, 42, 89, 97, 106, 130, 138–9, 145, 154, 177, 186, 242
eyeliner, 27, 42, 50, 80, 84, 99, 103, 111, 132, 145, 150, 170, 177, 191, 222, 234

face wash, 7, 30, 90, 106, 149, 159, 185, 188, 195, 203, 233
facial, 17, 61, 68, 77, 84, 160–1, 170, 178, 229, 236, 243
Felix, Allyson, 190–3, 192
fitness. See diet and fitness
foundations, 8, 15–6, 22, 36, 50, 54–5, 75, 77, 89, 97, 108–9, 120, 135, 141, 143, 145, 147, 150, 156, 165, 167, 169, 177, 179, 182, 196, 198, 222, 241
fragrance, 5, 7, 11, 16, 24, 31, 38, 39, 42, 46, 47, 50, 60–61, 63, 65, 68, 76, 77, 80, 81, 85, 87, 92, 98, 99, 102, 108, 112, 113, 120, 126, 127, 131, 132, 136, 141–2, 146, 147, 149, 151, 154, 160, 161, 166, 167, 170, 171, 177, 182, 188, 189, 192, 193, 196, 198, 204, 210, 218,

219, 222, 224, 230, 231, 234, 237, 242–3, 243, 246, 247, 248, 252, 253
French beauty products, 157

Gilmore, Stephanie, *33*, 34–9, 37
Goulding, Ellie, 44–7, *157*

hair oil, 8, *13*, 154, 210, 212
hair color, *12*–3, 90, 98, 108, 112, 132, 225, 242, 246, 248
hair cut, 17, 46, 48, 90, 170, 224–5
hairstylists, 199–201, 213–15, 216–19. See also colorists
highlighters, 28, 55, 90, 153, 163, 166–7, 207, 218, 222, 229–30

Jenner, Kylie, 88–92

Kargman, Jill, 168–71
Kendrick, Anna, 7–11, 19
Kent, Julie, 82–7, 86
Keys, Madison, 220–5, 223
Kravitz, Zoë, 158–61, 249
Kruger, Diane, 202–6, 214, *249*

laser medicine, 238–9
Lewis, Juliette, *19*, 96, 96–9, *109*
lip product, 7–8, 11, 16, *19*, 22, 26–7, 28, *33*, 35–6, 42–3, 45, 50–1, 58, 64, 68, 75, 77, 80–1, 84, 89, 97, 99, 103, 107, 112, 120, 126, 130, 135–6, 141, 143, 145, 147, 150, 160–1, 170, 177, 182, 186, 191, 193, 196, 198, 204, 210, 212, 217, 219, 222, 224, 234, 242–3, 246–7, *249*, 251
lip treatment, 92
Lyons, Jenna, 40–43

Macpherson, Elle, 66–69
makeup artists, 26–7, 54–55, 70–2, 93–5, 116, *138–9*, 162–3
mascaras, 8, 16, 22, 28, 36, 42, 50, 58–9, 64, 68, *73*, 75, 77, 80, 84–5, 89, 103, 108, 120, 127, 135, 137, 145, 147, 150, 154, 156, 161, 165, 182–3, 186, 191, 196, 210, 212, 217, 222, 230, 241, 251
massage, 17, 24, 31, 43, 53, 64, 68, 80, 98, 108, 120, 136, 170, 178, 189, 192, 196, 204, 218, 119, 243, 248, 252
moisturizer, 7, 11, 15, 16, 18, 22, 30, 36, 41, 50, 57, 64, 76, 79, 84–5, 90, 98, 10, 125, 127, 129, 141, 146, 149, 154, 160–1, 181, 185–6, 191, 193, 195, 203–4, 221, 226
Monroque, Shala, 194–8, 197

nails, 17, 39, 43, 46–7, 61, 77, 92, 102, 120,

126, 133, 142, 146, 150, 170, 178, 192, 218, 225, 230, 136, 248

Paltrow, Gwyneth, 208–12, 211

Ratajkowski, Emily, 28–32
Richie, Nicole, *19*, 124–27, 125
Ringwald, Molly, 244–48, 249
Roberts, Emma, 118–22, 121
Roy, Rachel, 78–81

St. Vincent, 184–9, 199
services, 8, 9, 17, 24, 31, 43, 46–47, 53, 61, 64, 68, 77, 80, 87, 90, 92, 98, 102, 108, 112, 120–21, 126, 132–33, 136, 142, 146, 150, 154–5, 160–61, 166, 170, 178, 182, 189, 192, 196–97, 204, 209, 218, 225, 230, 236, 243, 248, 252–3
shampoo and conditioner, 8, 11, 16, 24, 31, 33, 36, 38, 42–3, 46, 51, 64, 68–9, 76, 87, 90, 98, 108, 112–3, 120, 124, 127, 131–2, 136, 146, 150, 160–1, 166–7, 170–1, 177, 182, 192–3, 196, 204, 210, 223, 248, 252
Shawkat, Alia, 207
Sierota, Sidney, 228–31
skin, camera-ready, *54*–5, *238–9*
skin care, 7–8, 11, 15–16, 18, 22, 24, 28, 30–3, 35–36, 38, 41–2, 43, 45–6, 47, 50, 51, *54*–5, 57–8, 59, 63, 65, 67–8, 69, 76, 77, 79, 81, 84, 85, 90, 91, 98, 99, 101, 103, 106, 107, 111, 113, 119, 122, 124–5, 127, 129–30, 131, 135–36, 137, 141, 145–6, 149, 151, 153, 156, 157, *157*, 159, 161, 165, 167, 169, 171, 175, 177, 179, 181–2, 183, 185, 188, 191, 195–6, 198, 203, 206, 209–10, 212, 217, 219, 221–2, 224, 229, 231, 233–4, 237, 241, 245, 247, 251–2, 253

Snow, Brittany, 240–43
Souza, Karla, 104–9
Stewart, Martha, 14–18, *73*
sunscreen, 7–8, 22, 35, 63, 90, 106, 119, 136, 165, 191, 203, 206, 209, 221, 226, 229, 241, 246, 251–2

Toledo, Isabel, 148–51, *249*

Union-Wade, Gabrielle, *19*, 232–7, 235

Vodianova, Natalia, 110–4, 114

Weiss, Emily56–61, 60, *157*
Wek, Alek, *19*, 20–5, 23

Zhu Zhu, 174–9, 176

Editor: Holly Dolce
Designer: Sebit Min
Design Manager: Devin Grosz

Library of Congress Control Number: 2016961377

ISBN: 978-1-4197-2666-8

Text © 2017 *The New York Times*
Principal photography copyright © 2017 Elizabeth Lippman: 20, 23, 25, 49, 51, 52, 56, 59, 60, 62, 65, 104, 107, 128, 131, 133, 190, 192, 193, 216, 219, 228, 231, 240, 243
Elizabeth Lippman for *The New York Times*: 29, 30, 32, 82, 85, 86, 88, 91, 92, 152, 155, 156
Erin Baiano for *The New York Times*: 74, 77, 79, 81, 125, 127, 164, 167, 168, 171, 194, 197, 198, 244, 247
Emily Berl for *The New York Times*: 9, 10, 96, 99, 158, 161
Yana Paskova for *The New York Times*: 40, 43, 148, 151
Dmitry Kostyukov for *The New York Times*: 103, 110, 113, 114
Karsten Moran for *The New York Times*: 14, 17, 18
Paul van Kan for *The New York Times*: 34, 37, 38
Jennifer S. Altman for *The New York Times*: 118, 121, 122
Andrew Testa for *The New York Times*: 174, 176, 179
Ben Sklar for *The New York Times*: 184, 187, 188
Guia Besana for *The New York Times*: 202, 205, 206
Damon Winter for *The New York Times*: 208, 211, 212
Melissa Lyttle for *The New York Times*: 220, 223, 224
Barbara P. Fernandez for *The New York Times*: 232, 235, 237
Tony Cenicola for *The New York Times*: 11, 69
Lauren Fleishman for *The New York Times*: 44, 47
Alexi Hobbs for *The New York Times*: 134, 137
Taylor Glascock for *The New York Times*: 140, 143
Joe Buglewicz for *The New York Times*: 144, 147
Tom Jamieson for *The New York Times*: 180, 183
Sally Ryan for *The New York Times*: 250, 253
Winnie Au for *The New York Times*: 66
Kristin Vicari for *The New York Times*s: 100

Published in 2017 by Abrams, an imprint of ABRAMS. All rights reserved. No portion of this book may be reproduced, stored in a retrieval system, or transmitted in any form or by any means, mechanical, electronic, photocopying, recording, or otherwise, without written permission from the publisher.

Printed and bound in the United States
10 9 8 7 6 5 4 3 2 1

Abrams books are available at special discounts when purchased in quantity for premiums and promotions as well as fundraising or educational use. Special editions can also be created to specification. For details, contact specialsales@abramsbooks.com or the address below.

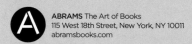

ABRAMS The Art of Books
115 West 18th Street, New York, NY 10011
abramsbooks.com